1: Russell Fork
2: Levisa Fork
3: Johns Creek
4: Big Sandy River
5: Little Sandy River
6: Tygarts Creek
7: Licking River
8: N. Fork Licking River
9: S. Fork Licking River
10: Hinkston Creek
11: Stoner Creek
12: Kentucky River
13: Eagle Creek
14: Elkhorn Creek
15: Benson Creek
16: Gilbert Creek
17: Jessamine Creek
18: Dix River
19: Hickman Creek
20: Silver Creek
21: Tates Creek
22: Boone Creek
23: Calloway Creek
24: Lower Howard Creek
25: Otter Creek
26: Fourmile Creek
27: Muddy Creek
28: Red River
29: S. Fork Kentucky River River
30: Red Bird River

31: M. Fork Kentucky River River
32: N. Fork Kentucky River River
33: Cumberland River
34: Big S. Fork Cumberland River
35: Little S. Fork Cumberland River
36: Rock Creek
37: N. Fork Cumberland River
38: Buck Creek
39: Rockcastle River
40: Laurel River
41: Salt River
42: Rolling Fork
43: Beech Fork
44: Floyds Fork
45: Plum Creek
46: Green River
47: Panther Creek
48: Pond River
49: Rough River
50: Mud River
51: Barren River
52: Gasper River
53: Drakes Creek
54: Nolin River
55: Little Barren River
56: Russell Creek

57: Tradewater River
58: Tennessee River
59: Clarks River
60: Bayou du Chien
61: Obion Creek
62: Mayfield Creek
63: Ballard Wildlife Management Area
64: Red River (Logan County)
65: Harrods Creek
66: Little Kentucky River

50 miles
50 kilometers

Freeway	Highway	Minor road

Unpaved road	Railroad	Borderline

Park/forest	Lake/river/creek

A Access point   **/** Dam   **) (** Tunnel

▲ Campground   **●** General point of interest   Waterfall

Cascades/rapids

CANOEING & KAYAKING
KENTUCKY

6TH EDITION

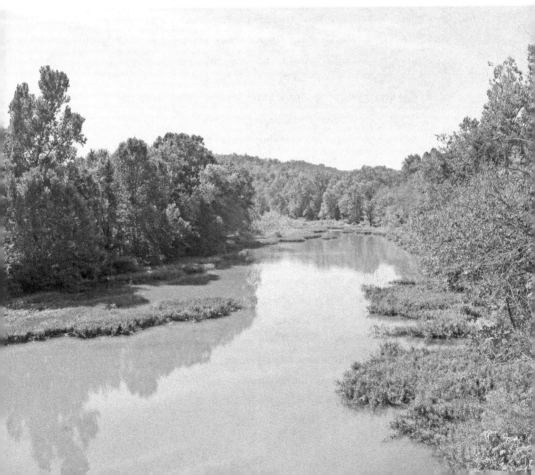

CANOEING & KAYAKING
KENTUCKY

6TH EDITION

BOB SEHLINGER
AND
JOHNNY MOLLOY

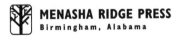
MENASHA RIDGE PRESS
Birmingham, Alabama

DEDICATION

THIS BOOK IS FOR ALL THE PADDLERS OF KENTUCKY—*from those on the waters of Land Between the Lakes, to the steep creeks of central Kentucky, to the casual floaters on the Licking, to the float fishermen on the Green, to the canoe campers on the Big South Fork, to those floating the entire length of the Kentucky River, to those on the Elkhorn on a Sunday afternoon—may you keep on stroking in the Bluegrass.*

Canoeing & Kayaking Kentucky

Copyright © 2017 by Bob Sehlinger and Johnny Molloy
All rights reserved
Published by Menasha Ridge Press
Distributed by Publishers Group West
Printed in the United States of America
Sixth edition, first printing

Cartography: Scott McGrew and Johnny Molloy
Cover design: Scott McGrew
Text design: Alian Design; adapted by Annie Long
Cover photo: Alexey Stiop / Alamy Stock Photo; interior photos: © Johnny Molloy, except as noted
Copy editor: Kerry J. Smith
Proofreader: Laura Franck
Indexer: Rich Carlson

Library of Congress Cataloging-in-Publication Data

Names: Sehlinger, Bob, 1945– author. | Molloy, Johnny, 1961– author. | Sehlinger, Bob, 1945–
    Canoeing and kayaking guide to Kentucky.
Title: Canoeing & kayaking Kentucky / Bob Sehlinger and Johnny Molloy.
Other titles: Canoeing and kayaking guide to Kentucky | Canoeing and kayaking Kentucky
Description: Sixth edition. | Birmingham, AL : Menasha Ridge Press, [2017]
    "Distributed by Publishers Group West" —T.p. verso. | Includes index.
Identifiers: LCCN 2016047129| ISBN 9781634040501 (paperback) | ISBN 9781634040518 (ebook)
    ISBN 9781634042093 (hardcover)
Subjects: LCSH: Canoes and canoeing—Kentucky—Guidebooks. | Kayaking—Kentucky—Guidebooks.
    White-water canoeing—Kentucky—Guidebooks. | Outdoor recreation—Kentucky—Guidebooks.
    Kentucky—Guidebooks.
Classification: LCC GV776.K4 S43 2017 | DDC 797.12209769—dc23
LC record available at https://lccn.loc.gov/2016047129

 MENASHA RIDGE PRESS
An imprint of AdventureKEEN
2204 First Avenue S., Suite 102
Birmingham, AL 35233
800-443-7227, fax 205-326-1012

Visit **menasharidge.com** for a complete list of our books and for ordering information. Contact us at our website, at **facebook.com/menasharidge**, or at **twitter.com/menasharidge** with questions or comments. To find out more about who we are and what we're doing, visit **blog.menasharidge.com**.

DISCLAIMER Paddling is an assumed-risk sport. The decision to run a river can be made only after an on-the-spot inspection, and a run should not be attempted without proper equipment and safety precautions. Neither Menasha Ridge Press nor the authors are responsible for any personal or property damage that may result from your activities. While every effort has been made to insure the accuracy of this guidebook, river and road conditions, along with phone numbers, websites, and other information, can change greatly from year to year.

TABLE OF CONTENTS

(Continued)

TABLE OF CONTENTS *(Continued)*

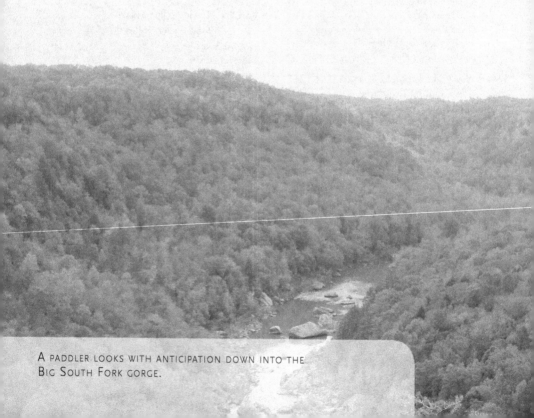

A PADDLER LOOKS WITH ANTICIPATION DOWN INTO THE
BIG SOUTH FORK GORGE.

ACKNOWLEDGMENTS

Thanks to all the people who helped with this sixth and latest edition of this guide, including my wife, Keri Anne. Thanks to Steve Spencer of the Western Kentucky University Outdoor Leadership Program for his help and photos. Thanks to Greg Woosley for helping with the Jessamine Creek and Hickman Creek write-ups. Dedicated paddlers like him strengthen whitewater boating all around. A special thanks to Barry Grimes and Don Spangler for helping us with much of the Kentucky whitewater from beginning to end and for offering insight into the ever-changing state of paddling. Thanks to American Whitewater and Scott Collins for their help, to Jim Thaxton for showing us around the Licking River watershed, to Ed Council for his help on the Elkhorn, to Alice Rankin for her help on Four Mile Creek, to Bradley Monton for his insight, and to Mark Branch for his paddling expertise. Thanks to my brothers for going canoeing with me on the Green, to Steve Grayson for paddling the South Fork Licking, and to John Cox for paddling in the Big South Fork. Thanks to Ben Culbertson for guiding us around the Red River Gorge. Also, thanks to all the folks at Menasha Ridge Press for making this book happen.

—*Johnny Molloy*

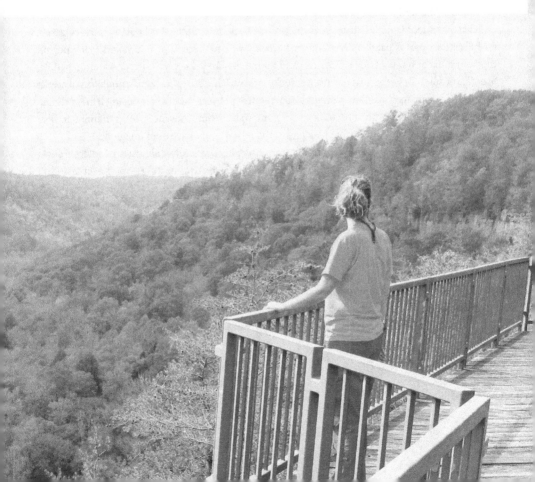

PREFACE

Welcome to the sixth edition of this guide covering paddling destinations in the Bluegrass State. We continue to update this book in order to make paddling adventures here in Kentucky easier. Canoeing and kayaking rival horses and basketball as a way of life for Kentuckians. Okay, that may be an exaggeration. Nevertheless, paddling the Bluegrass has a rabid following that increases on a yearly basis, and increases as more paddling destinations are opened, especially with the advent of state paddling trails. The first edition of this book, written by Kentucky native Bob Sehlinger, has become a classic and helped propel paddling to the forefront among outdoor enthusiasts throughout the commonwealth. Since 1978, untold Kentuckians have used continually updated editions of this book as a river resource. And as one paddler brought another one into the fold—passing down the paddle if you will—this book has been the standard, opening new rivers and streams to those who ventured forth with excitement that is only found when your boat curves around a new bend of a new stream offering new scenery and new opportunities. As Kentucky outdoor legend Arthur B. Lander Jr. wrote in the original introduction to this book, "drifting down a lazy, meandering river, or maneuvering a canoe or kayak through a jumble of boulders on a roller coaster of whitewater, is not only great fun, but a genuine mental and physical challenge. Americans are adventuresome by character, and are quick to seek the exhilaration that only life in the outdoors can bring."

That statement is no less true today than it was back then. Since this book was first released, a whole new class of paddlers has emerged. Today we have recreational kayakers, each person captaining his or her boat down streams. And then there are those ply SUPs, or stand-up paddleboards, yet another way to float down a Kentucky stream. The "steep creekers" paddle small creeks with limited drainages that flow perhaps a dozen times per year, taking hair-raising trips and challenging the heretofore limits of the Kentucky whitewater realm. Advances and variations in boat designs have gone far beyond what paddlers of the 1970s could have even imagined.

Today we have modern kayaks ranging from tiny play boats for whitewater paddlers frolicking in rapids to sit-on-top recreational kayaks to longer touring boats. Despite decreasing in popularity, canoes have come a long way too. State-of-the-art varied plastic composites range from heavily rockered whitewater boats to long-and-deep touring boats designed for extended trips to single-person boats for both whitewater and casual streams.

This book attempts to inform paddlers of paddling opportunities in the Bluegrass State, especially as the sport has advanced and many new streams are being explored. New watercourses have been added to this latest edition. We have also added GPS coordinates for all the put-ins and take-outs on the paddling routes, thereby allowing you to use your GPS guidance system or smartphone to make your paddling adventures easier. This guidebook is the product of scouting miles of river, and hours of map work and research writing. Along the way, many memories were made. We hope you will make some memories of your own, paddling the streams of Kentucky.

USING THIS GUIDE

First, a brief **overview** introduces each river profiled in this guide.

Second, a list of **topographic maps** that can be used for a particular section of river is provided. Topo maps are listed in the order in which the river flows. Unless otherwise noted, all maps are located on the Kentucky Index of the United States Geological Survey (USGS). Topos are available at outdoors and sporting-goods stores, at many public libraries, and online (in both digital and hard-copy formats) at websites including store.usgs.gov, topozone.com, and mytopo.com. A number of online sources, including the USGS, offer topos at no cost as well as for purchase.

Third, the river segment profiled is in most cases labeled and identified by the section **put-in,** followed by the section **take-out.** For example, the first segment of the Russell Fork is Bartlick Bridge to Garden Hole (page 13). Note that a few paddles are loops or out-and-back routes; thus, they have a single access point.

Fourth, an **at-a-glance box** lists basic river data, including class, gauge, level, gradient, and scenery.

Class, or river difficulty, has been adapted from a system developed by American Whitewater and is rated Class I–VI. For detailed information on the rating system, see Appendix A (pages 238–239).

Gauge indicates whether the method of gauging the river is visual, obtained by phone, or obtained online. If the gauge is visual, you literally have to look at the river to determine whether it is runnable or not.

Level indicates the flow rates at which a particular river can be run. Each section of river has its own personality when it comes to "too high" or "too low." A useful range is indicated by a comfortable minimum and a reasonable maximum flow rate. Rivers can be run at much higher levels by experts who know them well and at significantly lower levels by determined rock bashers who do not mind wading and lifting over shallow places. "N/A" means that a specific number is unavailable. Government agencies like the USGS measure river flows at gauging stations throughout the country. This information is collected and recorded hourly. You will find websites and phone numbers listed in the discussion of river gauges following. You will also encounter "paddler's gauges" painted on bridge piers and rocks; although not reported on websites, they are used by many canoeists and kayakers.

Gradient is the average drop of the river in feet per mile. For example, 2 means that the river drops at an average rate of 2 feet per mile. Note that the difficulty of a river's rapids is not determined only by gradient. Some rivers drop evenly over continuous rapids of roughly the same difficulty; others alternate between long pools and drops that are steeper than the gradient would indicate. Waterfalls are an extreme example of this. Geological peculiarities, such as huge boulders, high ledges, and gorges must also be considered. The accompanying river descriptions will give some insight.

Scenery is ranked on an A–D scale: A indicates remote wilderness areas with little sign of civilization; B indicates more-settled (but still beautiful) pastoral countryside; C indicates lots of development (cities or industrial areas); and D, unfortunately, indicates pollution, rundown buildings, and other forms of landscape abuse. The quality of the scenery along a river often changes. For example, the Green River within Mammoth Cave National Park is considered B, even A at times, but becomes C on its lower reaches, where barges are common.

Fifth, a **Description** of the specific section of the river is provided.

Sixth, **Shuttle** lists detailed driving directions to both the put-in and the take-out. (Loops and out-and-back routes require no shuttling and are designated instead with "Directions.")

Seventh, **Gauge** shows which gauges are needed to determine river runnability. Again, note that gauges are not available for some streams.

Finally, **maps** detail each river included in this guidebook. They include put-ins, take-outs, and mileage segments, plus features of interest such as bridges, landing areas, rapids, and confluences with other rivers, creeks, and streams. These maps will aid you in finding your way, but they are no substitute for detailed USGS topographic maps, public-land maps, or digital maps.

USING RIVER GAUGES

The Water Resources Division of the USGS measures water flows on most rivers in the United States at frequent intervals; The US Army Corps of Engineers and various power companies collect similar information. These flows are recorded in cubic feet per second (cfs) and are available to everyone.

The key variable is the height of the river at a fixed point. Gauge houses, situated on most rivers, consist of a well at the river's edge with a float attached to a recording clock. The gauge reads in hundredths of feet. Rating tables are constructed for each gauge to get a cfs reading for each level.

This information is very useful for paddlers who are planning a trip. In the "old days," paddlers had to phone various government offices and listen to recorded messages. They also contacted outfitters and private individuals who kept track of nearby paddler gauges. Nowadays we can get this information quickly at various websites, along with the weather! A few clicks gather information that would have taken us dozens of phone calls to obtain. Multiple websites provide backup when a single site goes down.

WATER-LEVEL SITES

USGS

Real-time water levels for Kentucky can be found at waterdata.usgs.gov/ky/nwis/rt. At this in-depth website, hundreds of gauges for the entire country are updated continually, and graphs showing recent flow trends are now available at the touch of a mouse. This is the greatest thing for paddlers since dry bags were invented.

AMERICAN WHITEWATER

This website collects USGS gauge readings for whitewater rivers throughout the country and automatically extrapolates water levels on rivers not covered by these gauges. They have an individual section for Kentucky's streams, americanwhitewater.org/content/River/state -summary/state/KY, that will prove very valuable to paddlers in the Bluegrass State, and can be accessed through any smartphone.

WATERLINE SERVICE

Waterline is a free, 24-hour phone service covering most of the USGS gauges mentioned in this book. Their figures are continuously updated every few hours, 24 hours a day, 7 days a week. They can be accessed by phone, without a computer. This is very useful when you have limited reception and can't get on the Internet.

To get a reading, call 800-452-1737. This gets you into an automated menu; you then dial the code number of the river gauge you want. You will get the current reading and a number of prior readings. For more information, call Waterline at 800-945-3376 or check their website at h2oline.com for the site codes of the river and streams about which you are interested.

RATING RIVER DIFFICULTY

American Whitewater's River Classification System (see Appendix A, pages 238–239) provides a good framework for discussing river difficulty. However, there are considerable variations in how this system is interpreted nationwide. Some expert paddlers tend to underrate everything, and an inexperienced paddler may go the other way and overestimate the difficulty. What seems horrendous to one person may be quite manageable to a more skilled paddler. If you have any doubts about your ability to handle a run, talk to paddlers who have done it before or allow some extra time to scout.

For years, there has been pressure to downgrade rivers in response to innovations in boat design and technique. We have chosen not to do this; thus, some rivers and creeks in this guide may seem overrated to expert paddlers. However, do not expect to finesse a "steep creek" like Lower Howards Creek

because you have run Russell Fork a few times! Every year, a number of steeper, more demanding runs are being run and redefine the limits of whitewater sport.

PADDLER SAFETY AND RIGHTS

HAZARDS AND SAFETY

Hazardous situations likely to be encountered on rivers and creeks must be identified and understood for safe paddling. The lure of high adventure, especially on little-run streams, has in part explained why there are so many more paddlers these days. Unfortunately, an alarming number were not prepared for what they encountered and lost their lives. They didn't use good judgment or just didn't understand the potential dangers. Below are some safety guidelines.

WINTER PADDLING

Winter paddling can be beautiful, but it can also be when the steep creeks are running high, which can make it quite dangerous unless certain precautions are taken. Some rules that should be followed by boaters are as follows:

1. Paddle those streams on which you can walk to shore at any point. It is best to stay off the larger rivers and those nearing flood stage.

2. Always have at least three boats in the party.

3. Everyone should have a complete change of clothing in a waterproof container that will withstand pressures of immersion.

4. Each paddler should carry on his person a supply of matches in a waterproof container.

5. Remember that the classification of any particular river is automatically upgraded when canoeing in cold weather. This is due to the extreme effects on the body upon immersion in cold water.

COLD-WEATHER SURVIVAL

With more and more paddlers going out in the cold weather to engage in their sport, a basic knowledge of cold-water and cold-weather survival is necessary. When immersed in water, the loss of heat from the body becomes much more rapid, and survival times without suitable clothing in cold water become very short. For instance, wet clothes lose about 90% of their insulating value and lose heat 240 times faster than dry clothing.

The following table gives the approximate survival times of humans immersed in water at various temperatures.

Water Temp (°F)	Exhaustion or Unconsciousness	Survival Time
32.5	0–15 min.	0–45 min.
32.5–40	15–30 min.	30–60 min.
40–50	30–60 min.	1–3 hrs.
50–60	1–2 hrs.	1–6 hrs.
60–70	2–7 hrs.	2–40 hrs.
70–80	3–12 hrs.	3 hrs.–?

The greatest change in survival time occurs as the water temperature drops below 50 degrees.

Swimming in cold water increases the flow of water past the body, pumping heat out of the clothing so that heat production is outpaced by heat loss. If there is no prospect of getting out of the water immediately, survival time will be longer if one does not swim but relies on a life jacket for flotation. Better still, assume the HELP position (Heat Escape Lessening Position) in which the knees are tucked close to the chest. This allows one to retain body heat longer. It is, therefore, imperative that a life jacket with adequate flotation be worn. Swim only if there is danger downstream.

A number of new materials have been developed that make cold-weather paddling more comfortable and certainly safer. Materials such as polypropylene, pile, and fleece tend to wick wetness away from the body and dry very quickly. Wool has the ability to provide warmth when wet, but the newer materials do it better. Worn under a paddling jacket and pants, they can be very effective. For the decked boater who is more likely to get wet, a wet or dry suit is highly recommended. Also, a polypro or wool cap can help tremendously because a great deal of body heat is lost through an unprotected head or neck.

Dry clothing should definitely be carried in a waterproof bag on all winter trips and changed into if one gets wet. Quite often, you must insist that the victim change clothing and render assistance in changing because of his lack of coordination. The victim more than likely will be totally unaware of his poor reactions.

Symptoms of exposure occur generally as follows: uncontrollable shivering; vague, slow, slurred speech; memory lapses; slowing of reactions, fumbling hands, and apparent exhaustion. Unconsciousness will follow and then death. The mental effects will be similar to those observed in states of extreme fatigue.

In cases of extreme exposure, build a fire and give the victim a warm drink, if he is able to swallow; strip him and put him into a sleeping bag with another person who is also stripped. Remember that the victim must be warmed from an outside heat source since he cannot generate his own body heat. Do not give the victim any form of alcohol.

KNOWING YOUR RIGHTS ON THE RIVER

The definition of a "navigable" stream is open to discussion. The term is not clear and its interpretation has sparked controversy all across the country. In Kentucky, a navigable stream is one that can support either commercial or recreational boating. That covers a lot of water—the commercial classification meaning specifically barge traffic, the recreational aspect connoting powerboats, canoes, kayaks, rafts, houseboats, and so on. It's a broad, debatable term, especially in the eyes of the mining industry, which cannot pollute navigable waters without being fined. Attempts have been made in the past to protect all waterways from flagrant pollution, but the measure met with defeat in the state legislature due to heavy opposition from mining lobbyists. However, in 2014, the state upgraded water quality standards when permitting mines into waterways.

The paddler's right to run rivers, all of which are "in the public domain," is guaranteed in Kentucky statutes. Landowners' rights to prohibit trespassing on their land along creeks, if they so desire, are also guaranteed. Therefore, access to rivers must be secured at highway rights-of-way or on publicly owned lands if permission to cross privately owned lands cannot be secured. In granting you access to a river, landowners are extending a privilege to you as they extend such to hunters who stop by their doors and seek permission to shoot doves in their cornfields. Don't betray landowners' trust if they extend to you the privilege to camp or launch canoes or kayaks from their riverbanks. Don't litter, drive through newly planted fields, or forget to close gates. Tenure of land, landholding, and the right to do with it what you want, is serious business to landowners. Some farmers can't accept the concept of "land stewardship" ascribed to by many city paddlers today. They don't feel any compulsion or responsibility toward the paddling community and their pursuit of legal rights. In some cases, they might even resent people driving hundreds of miles for the pleasure of floating down a river. They may even feel that they "own" the river you want to paddle.

On the other hand, it may be that the landowner you seek permission from is intrigued with paddling and will be quite friendly and approachable. Value this friendship and don't give cause to deny you access to the river at some time in the future.

Paddlers are trespassing when they portage, camp, or even stop for a lunch break, if they disembark from their boats on the water. If you are approached by a landowner when trespassing, by all means be cordial and understanding and explain your predicament (in the case of a portage or lunch break). Never knowingly camp on private land without permission. If you do encounter a perturbed landowner, don't panic. Keep cool and be respectful.

Landowners certainly have the right to keep you off their land, and the law will side with them unless they inflict harm upon you, in which case they may be both civilly and criminally liable. If you threaten a landowner verbally, and physically move toward him or her with apparent will to do harm, he or she has all the rights of self-defense and can protect himself or herself in accordance with the perceived danger that you impose. Likewise, if the landowner points a gun at you, fires warning shots, assaults, injures, or wounds you or a boater in your group, you are certainly in the right to protect yourself. The landowner has no right to detain you as if holding you for the sheriff. If you fear for your own life at the hands of the landowner, you do have the right to protect yourself.

The confrontations between belligerent paddlers and cantankerous landowners are to be avoided, that's for sure. Although the happenstance of such a meeting may be rare, paddlers nonetheless should know their rights, and the rights of landowners. Judges don't like trespassers any more than they like landowners who shoot trespassers.

THE DRAINAGES OF KENTUCKY

All the major rivers in Kentucky flow in a westerly, or northwesterly, direction. From east to west, the major rivers are the Big Sandy, Licking, Kentucky, Salt, Green, Tradewater, Cumberland, and Tennessee. They all empty into the Ohio River, which forms the northern boundary of Kentucky for 664 miles from Catlettsburg on the east to the Mississippi River on the west. About 97% of the total area of the commonwealth drains into the Ohio River.

The claim that Kentucky has more miles of running water than any state except Alaska is not unfounded; there are approximately 54,000 miles of streams and rivers when you add up all the major tributaries to the Ohio River, plus Mayfield Creek, Obion Creek, and Bayou du Chien, which drain into the Mississippi River in the far western Jackson Purchase region. The Tennessee River, which empties into the Ohio River at Paducah, is the fifth-largest river system in the United States, with a basin of more than 40,000 square miles occupying portions of seven states (1,055 square miles are in Kentucky alone). The Ohio River at its mouth is exceeded in volume of flow only by the lower Mississippi River. On the average, the Ohio River discharges three times more water than the upper Mississippi River, and about three and one-third times more water than the Missouri River. As a point of comparison, the Ohio's volume is about the same as both the Columbia and St. Lawrence rivers, major rivers of the North American continent.

The Cumberland and Green River basins both have considerably more square miles than any one of Kentucky's other five major basins. The Cumberland River basin drains more than 18,000 square miles in Kentucky and Tennessee. The river's headwaters are in extreme southeastern Kentucky (Poor Fork in Letcher County and Martins Fork in Bell County), and its mouth is at Smithland, in Livingston County of western Kentucky.

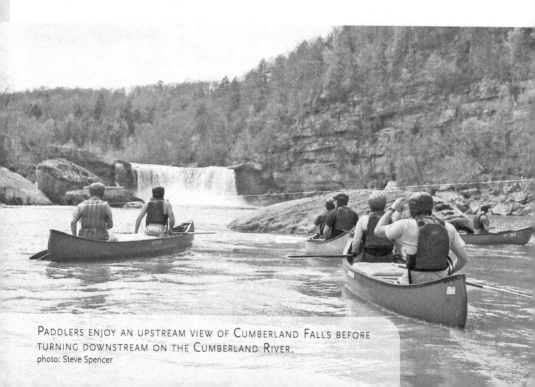

PADDLERS ENJOY AN UPSTREAM VIEW OF CUMBERLAND FALLS BEFORE TURNING DOWNSTREAM ON THE CUMBERLAND RIVER.
photo: Steve Spencer

Between the so-called "upper and lower" Cumberland basins, the river flows through Tennessee, where at least half of its basin lies. The Green River and its many tributaries flow across central Kentucky, encompassing more than 9,000 square miles of basin. In decreasing basin size are the Kentucky River, roughly 6,940 square miles; the Licking River, 3,670 square miles; the Salt River, 2,890 square miles; and finally the Big Sandy River basin at Kentucky's far eastern boundary with 2,280 square miles in Kentucky alone.

The quality of streams in Kentucky is generally good, although portions of several drainages are polluted by acid water and washings from coal mines, brine from oil fields, and sewage and industrial wastes. The situation has improved, since many mine sites have been reclaimed. The Levisa Fork of the Big Sandy River is basically a high-quality mountain stream. However, some mine drainage has made the water hard and high in sulfates. The upper Cumberland River also has high-quality water typical of a mountain stream, but it receives much less mine drainage and so is of better quality than the Levisa Fork. The Kentucky River drains a limestone area and is typical of many of Kentucky's streams; its water is hard and of the calcium bicarbonate type. The Tradewater River is an example of a small river that contains much acid from iron, manganese, and aluminum compounds, while Mayfield Creek is an example of the excellent water in the Jackson Purchase region.

In general, the water in small creeks in Kentucky is of the highest quality, especially in the mountains, but it is also the easiest to pollute because of the limited flows. Water in the large rivers, such as the Kentucky, Green, Tennessee, and Ohio, is more or less uniform in quality (or lack thereof) because the flows of these rivers tend to decrease the differences in the quality of the water entering from the tributaries.

Seasonal variations in the flow levels of watercourses are based on fluctuations in rainfall. Kentucky's yearly average of 46 inches of rain is equal to about 32 trillion gallons a year for all of Kentucky. About 37% of this, or 12 trillion gallons, runs either directly into the streams or through the ground and eventually into the streams. This much water alone would keep the Ohio River flowing for about 70 days at average flow. March and April are Kentucky's rainiest months. An average of 5.05 inches of precipitation a month falls in March, the rainiest month. October is the driest month, with an average of 2.35 inches of precipitation.

Mayfield Creek is in the Jackson Purchase region, a part of the state underlain with thick soils, sands, and gravels. Water stored in these materials during the winter and spring later seeps out to help maintain flow in hot, dry months. In the far eastern coalfield region, land slopes are steep, bedrock appears at the surface, and the soil is relatively thin. There is less opportunity and capacity for water storage in the ground.

Localized soil conditions have a great deal to do with stream flow, as do plant life, terrain slope, ground cover, and air temperature. In summer, during the peak growing season, water is used more readily by plants, and higher air temperatures encourage increased evaporation. The fall and winter low-water periods are caused by decreased precipitation, although since the ground is frozen and plant use of water is for the most part halted, abnormally high amounts of rain, or water from melting snow, can cause flash floods because surface runoff is high—there's no place for the water to go but into creeks and rivers. Though surface runoff is first to reach the river, it is groundwater that keeps many larger streams flowing during rainless periods. Drought can lower the water table drastically. Soil erosion is related to surface runoff—hilly land in intensive agricultural use is a prime target for loss of topsoil and flash flooding. The Salt River basin has severe soil erosion that creates continued and increasing chances of flooding. The Barren River basin, a tributary to the Green River, is intensely farmed, but the chance of flooding is less severe since the soil is absorbent and the terrain is relatively flat.

KENTUCKY WILD RIVERS SYSTEM

Nine Kentucky rivers of exceptional quality and aesthetic character are protected from development by the Wild Rivers System enacted by the Kentucky legislature. The rivers' rights-of-way—the linear corridor encompassing all visible land on each side of the river—are protected from strip mining, the construction of any impoundments, new roads, and buildings, or timber cutting within 2,000 feet of the middle of the watercourses. These wild rivers and their corridors add up to 114 river miles and 26,382 acres of land.

The nine rivers, six of which are classic paddling streams, are remote and as unspoiled as any in Kentucky, and have rocky cliffs, sweeping forests, and abundant fish and wildlife resources along their free-flowing paths. They are essentially untouched by the works of man, and are rich in recreational opportunity. Their protection is in the hands of Kentucky's Department for Natural Resources and Department for Environmental Protection.

Six of Kentucky's eight wild rivers are in the upper Cumberland basin, one is in the Kentucky River drainage, and one is in the Green River system. There is one wild river in each of Kentucky's two national parks and six in Daniel Boone National Forest (including one in a national geological area in the forest). The wild rivers and their boundaries are as follows:

◇ **CUMBERLAND RIVER** 6.1 miles, from Summer Shoals, in Whitley County, to the backwaters of Lake Cumberland, in McCreary and Whitley Counties.

◇ **RED RIVER** 9.1 miles, from the KY 746 bridge to the mouth of Swift Camp Creek, in the Red River Gorge Geological Area; in Wolfe and Powell Counties of the Stanton District of Daniel Boone National Forest.

◇ **ROCKCASTLE RIVER** 15.9 miles of whitewater, from the KY 1956 bridge to the backwaters of Lake Cumberland, in Pulaski and Laurel Counties.

◇ **GREEN RIVER** 26 miles in the confines of Mammoth Cave National Park; a classic flatwater run with camping allowed on islands or riverside sites, abundant wildlife, and rivers bubbling up from underground caverns.

◇ **BIG SOUTH FORK OF THE CUMBERLAND RIVER** 10.2 miles of one of the most celebrated whitewater runs in the eastern United States, from the Tennessee border to Blue Heron, in Whitley County.

◇ **ROCK CREEK** 18 miles of good rainbow trout stream, from the Tennessee border to the White Oak Junction bridge.

◇ **MARTINS FORK OF THE CUMBERLAND RIVER** 3.9 miles of shallow, unnavigable water extending from the eastern boundary of Cumberland Gap National Historical Park to KY 987. The headwaters of this crystal-clear, brook trout–stocked stream are in a grove of virgin hemlock trees.

◇ **LITTLE SOUTH FORK OF THE CUMBER-LAND RIVER** 10.4 miles, from the KY 92 bridge in the backwaters of Lake Cumberland, in Wayne and McCreary Counties.

◇ **BAD BRANCH** A nonpaddled tributary of the Poor Fork Cumberland River in Letcher County; the lowermost 3 miles of the stream before it feeds into Poor Fork.

The state has also established a Blue Water Trails system. Managed by Kentucky Department of Fish and Wildlife, the goal of the Blue Water Trails system is to provide "thorough information for paddlers to enjoy floating Kentucky streams without worry." All the streams sections are open to public use. Maps are available online showing put-ins, take-outs, and other important information, such as dams.

ENVIRONMENTAL CONCERNS

Water quality is an ever-important issue as Kentucky becomes more populated. Presenting a set of environmental guidelines for all paddlers sounds like preaching, but with the number of persons using our creeks and rivers today, it is indeed a valid point. Many of the streams listed in this guide flow through national parks and forests, state-owned forests and wildlife management areas, and privately owned lands that in some cases are superior in quality and aesthetics to lands under public ownership. It is the paddling community's responsibility to uphold the integrity of these lands and their rivers by exercising environmentally sound guidelines. Litter, fire scars, pollution from human excrement, and cutting live trees is unsightly and affects the land in a way that threatens to ruin the outdoor experience for everyone.

Keep in mind that litter and liquid pollutants often end up in streams by nonpaddlers. That piece of trash by the highway or oil from an auto leak flows into a stream during a storm and enters the watershed. It is our job to keep our waterways clean no matter where we are. While on the river, paddlers should pack out everything they packed in: all paper litter and such nonbiodegradable items as cartons, foil, plastic jugs, and cans. Help keep our waterways clean for those who follow. If you are canoe camping, leave your campsite in better shape than you found it. If you must build a fire, build it at an established site, and when you leave, dismantle rock fireplaces, thoroughly drown all flames and hot coals, and scatter the ashes. Never cut live trees for firewood. Use biodegradable soap, and dump all dishwater at least 100 feet away from watercourses.

RECOMMENDED RUNS

With thousands of miles of paddling possibilities in the Bluegrass State, it's sometimes hard to know where to begin. The following paddling recommendations will help you get started. Note that some of the runs are shorter segments within featured paddles.

NOVICE MOVING WATER RUNS

11 Licking River: Falmouth to Butler (p. 44)

46 Cumberland River from Wolf Creek Dam to the Tennessee Border: Wolf Creek Dam to KY 771 (p. 147)

49 Floyds Fork of the Salt River: Fisherville to Cane Run (p. 155)

52 Green River: Mammoth Ferry to Houchins Ferry (p. 168)

55 Drakes Creek: Confluence to US 231 Bridge (p. 176)

59 Tradewater River: KY 120 Bridge to KY 132 Bridge (p. 188)

65 Cumberland River North of Lake Barkley: Lake Barkley Dam to the Ohio River (p. 204)

75 Red River of Logan County: KY 1041 to TN 102 Bridge (p. 223)

CLASSIC WHITEWATER PADDLING RUNS

1 Russell Fork (p. 11)

17 Red River: Upper Red River (p. 74)

29 Elkhorn Creek: Forks of Elkhorn to Peaks Mill Road (p. 100)

31 Calloway Creek: Smith Fork to Kentucky River (p. 104)

38 North Fork of the Cumberland River: Cumberland Falls to Lake Cumberland (p. 124)

40 Rockcastle River: Howard Place Access to KY 192 (p. 131)

42 Big South Fork Gorge of the Cumberland River: Burnt Mill Bridge to Leatherwood Ford (p. 138)

SECLUDED RUNS

38 North Fork of the Cumberland River: Williamsburg to Cumberland Falls (p. 123)

40 Rockcastle River: KY 1956 to Howard Place Access (p. 131)

52 Green River: Dennison Ferry to Brownsville (p. 168)

53 Russell Creek: Russell Creek Road to Green River (p. 171)

58 Nolin River: Nolin River Dam to Houchins Ferry (p. 186)

GREAT PADDLES FOR CHILDREN

16 Kentucky River Below the Forks: Lock 8 to Camp Nelson (p. 67)

49 Floyds Fork of the Salt River: Creekside Access to Fisherville (p. 155)

52 Green River: Dennison Ferry to Mammoth Ferry (p. 168)

58 Nolin River: Nolin River Dam to Houchins Ferry (p. 186)

66 Tennessee River North of Kentucky Lake: Kentucky Lake Dam to Haddock Ferry Road (p. 206)

OVERNIGHT CAMPING TRIPS

40 Rockcastle River: Livingston to I-75 Bridge Access (p. 129)

43 Big South Fork Gorge of the Cumberland River: Leatherwood Ford to Blue Heron (p. 140)

43 Big South Fork Gorge of the Cumberland River: Blue Heron to Yamacraw (p. 142)

52 Green River: Green River Lake Dam Through Mammoth Cave National Park (p. 166)

69 Land Between the Lakes Paddle Route (p. 209)

LAKE PADDLES

3 Johns Creek: Dewey Lake (p. 21)

4 Little Sandy River: Grayson Lake Portion of Sandy Hook to Grayson Lake (p. 23)

23 Dix River: Herrington Lake Portion of Logantown to Herrington Lake (p. 90)

52 Green River: Green River Lake Portion of Liberty to Green River Lake (p. 164)

74 Ballard Wildlife Management Area (p. 221)

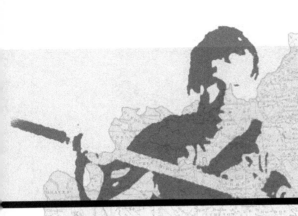
1 RUSSELL FORK

⟡ **OVERVIEW** Flowing out of Virginia and joined by the Pound River, the Russell Fork cuts a 1,600-foot gorge in the lonely Pine Ridge Mountains, forming what is referred to as the Great Breaks of the Pine Ridge. This incredible chasm with giant vertical walls and pounding whitewater bisects the Kentucky–Virginia border for several miles before plunging out of the mountains near Elkhorn City, Kentucky.

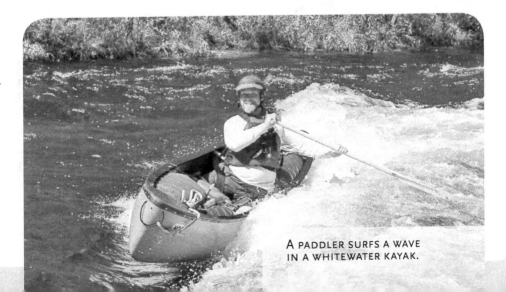

A PADDLER SURFS A WAVE IN A WHITEWATER KAYAK.

Russell Fork

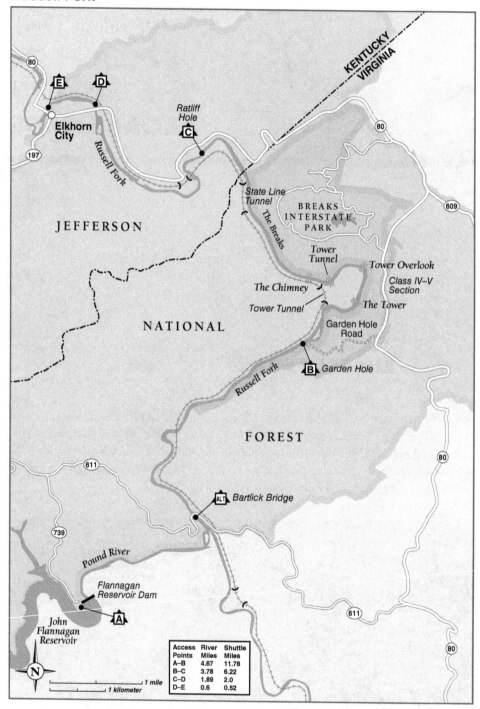

KENTUCKY
VIRGINIA

E

D

Ratliff
Hole

C

Elkhorn
City

Russell Fork

State Line
Tunnel

BREAKS
INTERSTATE
PARK

The Breaks

Tower
Tunnel

JEFFERSON

The Chimney

Tower
Overlook

*Class IV–V
Section*

Tower Tunnel

The Tower

NATIONAL

Garden Hole
Road

B Garden Hole

Russell Fork

FOREST

ALT Bartlick Bridge

Pound River

*Flannagan
Reservoir Dam*

A

*John
Flannagan
Reservoir*

N

	1 mile
	1 kilometer

Access Points	River Miles	Shuttle Miles
A–B	4.67	11.78
B–C	3.78	6.22
C–D	1.89	2.0
D–E	0.6	0.52

Before the 1990s, this river was seldom run but has since become a paddling mecca for whitewater enthusiasts from Kentucky, Virginia, and beyond, especially during the fall whitewater releases from the Flannagan Dam. The dammed Pound River joins the free-flowing Russell Fork at Bartlick, Virginia. From here, the river punches into a rugged gorge from the Garden Hole through the Breaks into Kentucky. The rapids ease up a bit beyond old Potters Ford, now known as Ratliff Hole, the first take-out beyond the gorge, before flowing into Elkhorn City.

For four October weekends, the Army Corps of Engineers draws down Flanagan Reservoir, releasing an average of 800–1,100 cfs into the Russell Fork, attracting paddlers from all over to tackle this beautiful and challenging waterway. The Russell Fork is a designated Kentucky Blue Water Trail.

◆ **MAPS** ELKHORN CITY, KY; DICKENSON, VA (USGS)

A Bartlick Bridge to Garden Hole

Class	II–III+
Gauge	Web
Level	Min. 400–Max. 1,500 (cfs)
Gradient	28'
Scenery	A

1A **DESCRIPTION** With the exception of fall water releases from Flannagan Dam (A), Bartlick Bridge (ALT) is the most commonly used upper access. This section becomes Class IV when the water is above 1,500 cfs. At normal water levels, this is a good intermediate run. In fall, paddlers start below Flannagan Dam, which adds 1.5 miles of water to the run. The put-in is in Virginia on the Pound River, below the dam, with easy Class II water on down to the confluence with the Russell Fork. Below the confluence, the gradient begins to increase, and the river broadens slightly to accommodate the additional volume. As canyon walls begin to rise on both sides, Garden Hole access (B) can be seen near the river's edge on the right. For anyone beginning to feel a little overwhelmed, this is the last chance to stop before entering the gorge.

◆ **SHUTTLE** From Elkhorn City, take KY/VA 80 East 7.8 miles into Virginia, then turn right on Garden Hole Road and follow it to the take-out. From the take-out, backtrack to VA 80, turn right, and continue east 4 miles to VA 611. Follow VA 611 for 3.3 miles to the put-in.

◆ **GAUGE** The gauge used for Russell Fork is a combination of two USGS gauges: Russell Fork at Haysi, VA, and Pound River below Flannagan Dam near Haysi, VA. Add the two and use the number to determine floatability. Minimum level is 400 cfs, maximum level is 1,500 cfs.

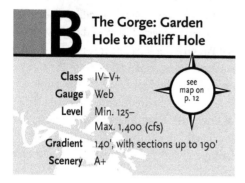

B The Gorge: Garden Hole to Ratliff Hole

Class	IV–V+
Gauge	Web
Level	Min. 125– Max. 1,400 (cfs)
Gradient	140', with sections up to 190'
Scenery	A+

see map on p. 12

1B DESCRIPTION At the Garden Hole, the drop increases markedly, and steep sandstone walls rise on both sides. The Russell Fork now pounds its way along a giant semicircular loop at the base of the mountain. Here, hidden by the shadows of the gorge, is a hellish continuum of thundering vertical drops and foam-blasted boulder gardens, where the river gradient reaches 190 feet per mile!

Many of the rapids in this section, including the consecutive 5-, 8-, and 9-foot vertical drops of Triple Drop; the awesome El Horrendo with drops of 10 and 15 feet, spaced only a boat length apart; and the boulder-strewn S-turn at Red Cliff had never been run before October 1976. This section is now run regularly but is still a solid Class V+. Needless to say, this section is for experts in top condition with bulletproof rolls.

Although scouting is not difficult, and portage routes around the major rapids are available, the rapids are intensely complex, technical, violent, and continuous. An upset in one of the milder rapids (Class III–IV) could lead to a nightmare swim through a Class V+ run. Dangers on this run, other than the obvious, include two long railroad tunnels on the left ridge that some paddlers risk walking through to facilitate scouting.

Beyond the loop, the river turns north and heads toward Elkhorn City, passing Ratliff Hole, the take-out for the gorge. Formerly known as Potters Ford, Ratliff Hole (C) has a steep road to tackle, but river access is excellent. This locale is a gathering spot for paddling enthusiasts, who trade tales of taming the now-famed whitewater that is Russell Fork.

◇ SHUTTLE From Elkhorn City, take KY 80 East 2.4 miles to the take-out. From the take-out, take KY 80 East 1.4 miles into Virginia and continue on VA 80 East 4 miles to turn right onto Garden Hole Road to the put-in.

◇ GAUGE The gauge used for Russell Fork is a combination of two USGS gauges: Russell Fork at Haysi, VA, and Pound River below Flannagan Dam near Haysi, VA. Add the two and use the number to determine floatability. Minimum level is 125 cfs, maximum level is 1,400 cfs.

≈≈≈

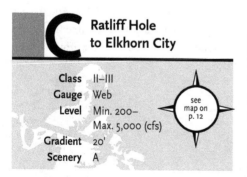

C Ratliff Hole to Elkhorn City

Class	II–III
Gauge	Web
Level	Min. 200– Max. 5,000 (cfs)
Gradient	20'
Scenery	A

see map on p. 12

1C DESCRIPTION This section starts at Ratliff Hole, formerly known as Potters Ford. This is the take-out for the gorge section of Russell Fork. Although primarily Class II rapids, the run does have one Class III. It is not normally run in open canoes but is used for training in play boats and rafts. These last two take-outs are in Elkhorn City.

✧ **SHUTTLE** From the intersection of KY 80 and KY 197 in Elkhorn City, take KY 197 (Russell Street) South just a short distance to the take-out on your right. To reach the put-in, backtrack to KY 80 and follow it east 2.4 miles to the put-in.

✧ **GAUGE** The gauge used for Russell Fork is a combination of two USGS gauges, Russell Fork at Haysi, VA, combined with Pound River below Flannagan Dam near Haysi, VA. Add the two together and use the number to determine floatability. Minimum level is 200 cfs,

maximum recommended level is 5,000 cfs. This combined gauge is posted on the American Whitewater Association website.

GPS COORDINATES		
ACCESS	**LATITUDE**	**LONGITUDE**
A	N37° 14.005'	W82° 20.676'
B	N37° 16.243'	W82° 18.177'
C	N37° 17.992'	W82° 19.276'
D	N37° 18.304'	W82° 20.567'
E	N37° 18.261'	W82° 21.141'

2 LEVISA FORK OF THE BIG SANDY RIVER

✧ **OVERVIEW** The Levisa Fork flows out of Virginia into Pike County in southeastern Kentucky, where it is impounded to form Fishtrap Lake. Below the lake, the Levisa Fork makes up one of the major drainages of eastern Kentucky as it flows through Floyd, Johnson, and Lawrence Counties before coming together with the Tug Fork to form the Big Sandy River. Runnable almost all year below the dam at Fishtrap Lake to its confluence with the Tug Fork, the Levisa Fork is big—averaging 80–110 feet in width. Civilization is continuous along the Levisa Fork, with a highway paralleling the stream on one side and a railroad on the other. Additionally, the Levisa Fork runs through the sizable communities of Pikeville, Paintsville, Prestonsburg, and Louisa. Amazingly, despite the overwhelming human presence, the Levisa Fork is not a total loss as a paddling stream. Sunk between deep banks that hide the bustle of civilization, the stream itself is tree lined and not at all unpleasant. Access is plentiful along its entire length, and the river is free of powerboat traffic, except for a small stretch in Lawrence County. Tall hills and bluffs (some man-made) make for pleasant viewing. The Levisa Fork's level of difficulty is Class I with occasional small shoals and rapids (Class I+). Dangers to navigation are limited to deadfalls (which are easily avoided), a man-made rapid below Louisa, and several low-water bridges. Difficulties also include a mud bottom and banks of soft sand that can easily swallow paddlers up to their waist if they step in the wrong place when putting in or taking out.

✧ **MAPS** MILLARD, PIKEVILLE, BROADBOTTOM, HAROLD, LANCER, PRESTONSBURG, PAINTSVILLE, OFFUTT, RICHARDSON, MILO, LOUISA (USGS)

Levisa Fork of the Big Sandy River: Fishtrap Lake Dam to Banner

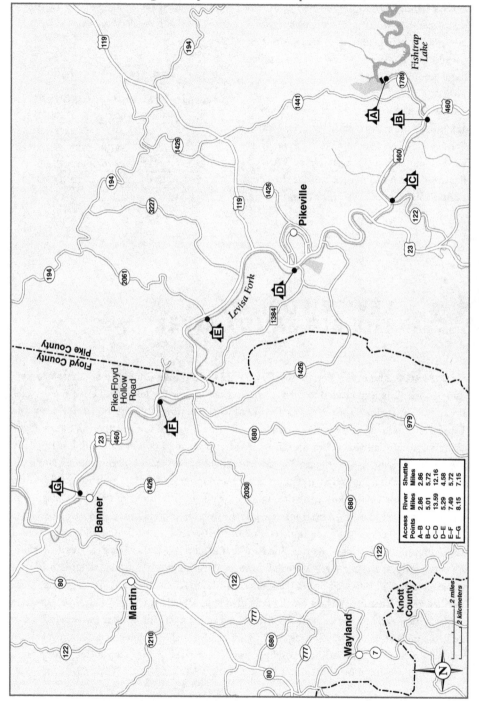

Access Points	River Miles	Shuttle Miles
A–B	2.86	2.86
B–C	5.01	5.72
C–D	13.59	12.16
D–E	5.29	4.58
E–F	7.49	5.72
F–G	8.15	7.15

A Fishtrap Lake Dam to Banner

Class	I (II)
Gauge	Web
Level	Min. 400–Max. flood (cfs)
Gradient	1.5'
Scenery	C

2A DESCRIPTION The river often flows clear from below Fishtrap Dam. It is 8 miles from the dam to KY 122, 13 miles from KY 122 to the north side of Pikeville, and 21 miles farther to Banner. Interestingly, the Levisa Fork of Big Sandy River formerly made a horseshoe-shaped loop in which the city of Pikeville rose. However, this bend through Peach Orchard Bottom flooded Pikeville all too often. Over 14 years a channel was cut through Peach Orchard Mountain, and the Levisa Fork rerouted one of the largest civil engineering projects in American history. The 8-mile segment immediately around Pikeville, including the rerouted channel, is a Kentucky Blue Water Trail.

⬦ SHUTTLE From Prestonsburg, take US 23 South to KY 1426 and the take-out in Banner. From Banner return to US 23 South and follow it 23 miles to veer right onto US 460 E/ Shelbiana Road. Follow it 5 miles, then split right to join KY 1441. Follow it 1.7 miles, then keep straight on KY 1789 for 1.2 miles to reach the put-in.

⬦ GAUGE The USGS gauge is Levisa Fork at Pikeville. Minimum reading should be 400.

GPS COORDINATES

ACCESS	LATITUDE	LONGITUDE
A	N37° 25.714'	W82° 24.863'
B	N37° 24.438'	W82° 26.417'
C	N37° 25.591'	W82° 29.930'
D	N37° 28.832'	W82° 32.686'
E	N37° 31.866'	W82° 34.687'
F	N37° 33.466'	W82° 38.057'
G	N37° 36.131'	W82° 42.015'

B Banner to Paintsville

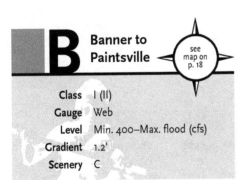

see map on p. 18

Class	I (II)
Gauge	Web
Level	Min. 400–Max. flood (cfs)
Gradient	1.2'
Scenery	C

2B DESCRIPTION The average width of the river here is 80–100 feet. It is 7 miles from Banner to the junction of KY 1428 and KY 194, and 13.5 miles farther to Auxier and the mouth of Johns Creek. It is 11 miles from Auxier to Paintsville. The boat ramp in Paintsville, off River Road near the confluence of Paint Creek and Levisa Fork, is a welcome treat for paddlers, who often have to forge their own carries on less floated rivers, such as the Levisa Fork.

⬦ SHUTTLE From Prestonsburg, take US 460/US 23 north 3.7 miles. Turn right onto KY 1428 and follow it 2.8 miles. Turn right onto Chessie Lane and follow it to curve right as it becomes River Road after 0.4 mile. Just after joining River Road, look left for the boat ramp in downtown Paintsville. To reach the

Levisa Fork of the Big Sandy River: Banner to Paintsville

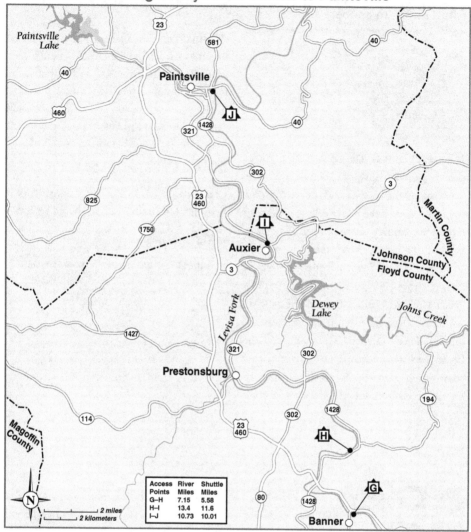

Access Points	River Miles	Shuttle Miles
G–H	7.15	5.58
H–I	13.4	11.6
I–J	10.73	10.01

put-in, backtrack to US 460/US 23 and follow it 15 miles to KY 1426 and the bridge over Levisa Fork at Banner.

◇ **GAUGE** The USGS gauge is Levisa Fork at Paintsville. The minimum reading should be 400.

GPS COORDINATES

ACCESS	LATITUDE	LONGITUDE
G	N37° 36.131'	W82° 42.015'
H	N37° 37.999'	W82° 42.031'
I	N37° 44.261'	W82° 45.270'
J	N37° 48.810'	W82° 47.485'

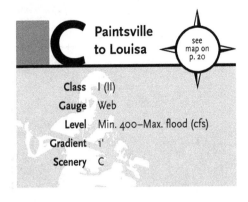

C Paintsville to Louisa

see map on p. 20

Class	I (II)
Gauge	Web
Level	Min. 400–Max. flood (cfs)
Gradient	1'
Scenery	C

 DESCRIPTION This section of river ranges from 80 to 110 feet wide. KY 581 offers nearly continuous scouting opportunities. It is 12 miles from Paintsville to the next access on KY 581, and 18 miles farther to the US 23 access near KY 1760. It is 17.5 miles from the US 23/KY 1760 access to downtown Louisa, where there is a boat ramp just off the town square, off Main Street, just before the Levisa Fork flows into the Big Sandy River.

SHUTTLE The take-out is at the Louisa boat ramp on Main Street in downtown Louisa, off Vinson Avenue. From the boat ramp in Louisa, turn left onto Vinson Avenue. After one block, turn right onto East Madison Street and follow it 0.4 mile. Turn left onto Old US 23 South and follow it 3.6 miles. Turn left onto US 23 South and follow it to Staffordsville. In Staffordsville, take KY 40 East into Paintsville, then turn left onto Mill Branch Road. Follow Mill Branch Road a short distance to veer right onto Broadway. Take Broadway a short distance to Depot Road. Turn left onto Depot Road, then make a quick right onto Chessie Lane. It soon turns to River Road, and shortly you will reach the boat ramp and put-in on the left.

GAUGE The USGS gauge is Levisa Fork at Paintsville. The minimum reading should be 400.

GPS COORDINATES

ACCESS	LATITUDE	LONGITUDE
J	N37° 48.810'	W82° 47.485'
K	N37° 51.603'	W82° 43.550'
L	N37° 56.343'	W82° 38.852'
M	N37° 59.371'	W82° 39.761'
N	N38° 1.250'	W82° 38.615'
O	N38° 4.863'	W82° 36.014'
P	N38° 6.995'	W82° 36.091'

3 JOHNS CREEK

OVERVIEW Johns Creek flows northwest out of Pike County into Dewey Lake and from there through Floyd County to empty into the Levisa Fork of the Big Sandy River south of Paintsville. Scenery on both sections consists of wooded hillsides and sandy banks with dense scrub vegetation.

MAPS PRESTONSBURG (USGS)

Levisa Fork of the Big Sandy River: Paintsville to Louisa

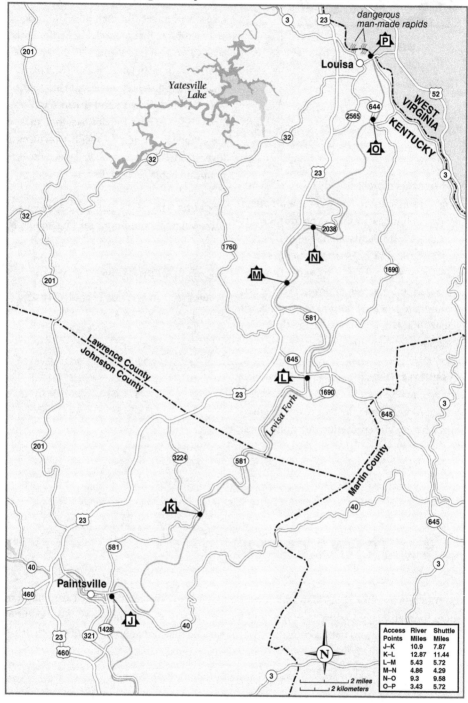

dangerous man-made rapids

Louisa

Yatesville Lake

WEST VIRGINIA

KENTUCKY

Lawrence County
Johnston County

Levisa Fork

Martin County

Paintsville

Access Points	River Miles	Shuttle Miles
J–K	10.9	7.87
K–L	12.87	11.44
L–M	5.43	5.72
M–N	4.86	4.29
N–O	9.3	9.58
O–P	3.43	5.72

2 miles
2 kilometers

KY 194 to Dewey Lake

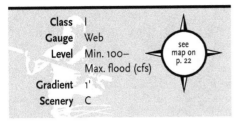

Class	I
Gauge	Web
Level	Min. 100–
	Max. flood (cfs)
Gradient	1'
Scenery	C

see map on p. 22

❖ DESCRIPTION The upper section from KY 194 to Dewey Lake can be run all year. Occasional logs border one side or another of the stream, which averages 20–30 feet wide above Dewey Lake. The upper section is almost devoid of current as a rule but is a passable paddle-camping run when combined with portions of Dewey Lake, a normally clear impoundment. Dewey Lake, bordered by Jenny Wiley State Park, has multiple access points, including roadside pulloffs. KY 194 runs along upper Johns Creek, offering scouting opportunities. Access to the upper section is plentiful and good.

❖ SHUTTLE From Prestonsburg, take KY 1428 East and turn left on KY 302. Follow KY 302 North 3 miles to Tom Wiley Road and the boat ramp take-out. To reach the put-in, backtrack on KY 302 South 3 miles to KY 1428. Turn left onto KY 1428 and travel south 3.8 miles. Turn left onto KY 194 and follow it east 12 miles to the bridge over Brushy Creek. The put-in is on your right at the confluence of Brushy and Johns Creeks.

❖ GAUGE The USGS gauge is Johns Creek near Meta, KY. The minimum reading should be 100 cfs.

GPS COORDINATES

ACCESS	LATITUDE	LONGITUDE
A	N37° 40.837'	W82° 35.348'
B	N37° 41.084'	W82° 39.166'
C	N37° 41.674'	W82° 43.589'
D	N37° 43.030'	W82° 43.313'
E	N37° 43.597'	W82° 44.568'

4 LITTLE SANDY RIVER

❖ OVERVIEW The Little Sandy River is born in southern Elliott County and flows northeast to the Ohio River through Carter and Greenup Counties.

❖ MAPS SANDY HOOK, ISONVILLE, BRUIN, WILLARD, GRAYSON, OLDTOWN, ARGILLITE, GREENUP (USGS)

Johns Creek

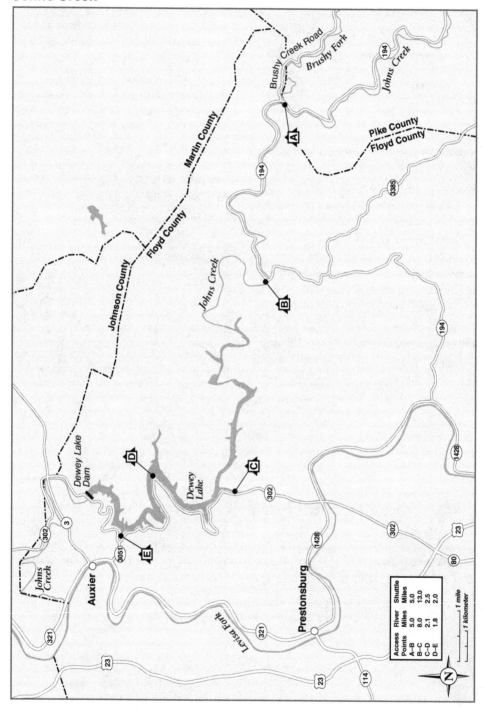

Access Points	River Miles	Shuttle Miles
A–B	5.0	5.0
B–C	8.0	13.0
C–D	2.1	2.5
D–E	1.8	2.0

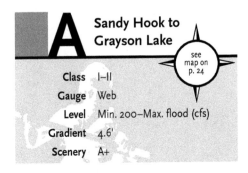

A
Sandy Hook to Grayson Lake

see map on p. 24

Class	I–II
Gauge	Web
Level	Min. 200–Max. flood (cfs)
Gradient	4.6'
Scenery	A+

4A **DESCRIPTION** From Sandy Hook (A) to the Dehart Road Bridge above Grayson Lake (B), the stream is runnable from January through April and following heavy rains at any time of year. A second bridge is not far downstream (C). This section is beautiful beyond belief, with exposed rock bluffs and overhangs and a luxurious forest of both evergreens and hardwoods. Interspaced along the river are flat terraces carpeted with lush bluegrass, perfect for camping. The Little Sandy flows over a bed of gravel and mud in this upper gorge section with frequent sandbars and small Class I+ rapids to make paddling interesting. The river's width is from 20 to 35 feet on average. Navigational hazards are primarily deadfalls washed into the gorge from above Sandy Hook.

From the KY 7 bridge, near its junction with KY 706, (D) downstream into Grayson Lake, the Little Sandy can be run all year thanks to the water backup from the lake pool. This section also runs through a gorge and is extremely scenic, with small waterfalls visible at adjoining feeder streams. Obviously, due to the backwash, the stream is wider here (75–80 feet), and there is no current. Access is good, and many take-outs are available according to how far into the lake you wish to paddle. This section is excellent for paddle camping, and there are no navigational hazards.

It is 11 miles from Sandy Hook to the KY 7 bridge near KY 706 and 15.5 miles farther to the Clifty Creek embayment (E) access on Grayson Lake at Grayson Lake Marina.

SHUTTLE To reach the lower access from Exit 172 on I-64, take KY 7 South. Stay with KY 7 over Grayson Lake Dam. Turn left just before the Clifty Creek embayment and a boat ramp on the right. If you reach South Clifty Access for the Grayson Lake Wildlife Management Area, you have gone a half mile too far and over the Clifty Creek embayment.

GAUGE The gauge is Little Sandy River at Grayson, KY. This gauge is below Grayson Lake and the creek paddling, so factor that in. The gauge should read at least 200 cfs.

GPS COORDINATES

ACCESS	LATITUDE	LONGITUDE
A	N38° 5.212'	W83° 7.452'
B	N38° 6.795'	W83° 7.074'
C	N38° 7.140'	W83° 6.323'
D	N38° 8.638'	W83° 4.083'
E	N38° 12.092'	W83° 0.673'
F	N38° 14.764'	W82° 59.200'

Little Sandy River: Sandy Hook to Grayson Lake

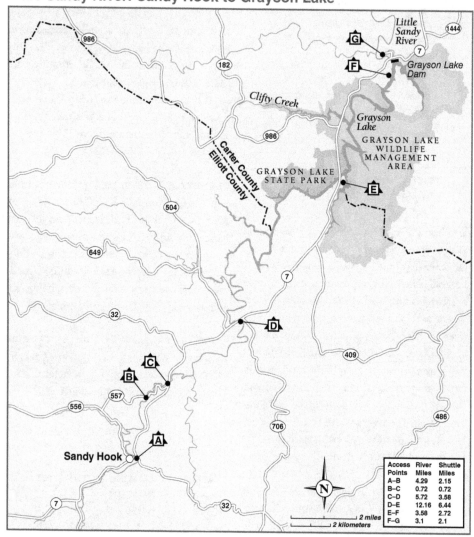

Access Points	River Miles	Shuttle Miles
A–B	4.29	2.15
B–C	0.72	0.72
C–D	5.72	3.58
D–E	12.16	6.44
E–F	3.58	2.72
F–G	3.1	2.1

B Grayson Lake Dam to Ohio River

Class	I–II
Gauge	Web
Level	Min. 150–Max. flood (cfs)
Gradient	1.6'
Scenery	A to B–

4B **DESCRIPTION** Below the Grayson Lake Dam, the Little Sandy continues to be extraordinary to the intersection of the KY 7 bridge near Leon (H). Small and intimate, the river once again averages 25–40 feet in width and flows beneath steep rock walls and overhangs on the west and forest (with some cultivated land) on the east. This section can be combined with a loop of the Jenny Wiley Trail,

Little Sandy River: Grayson Lake Dam to Ohio River

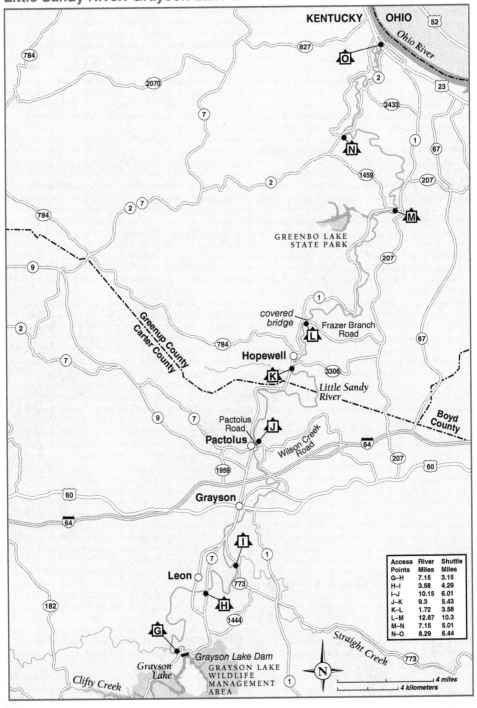

Access Points	River Miles	Shuttle Miles
G–H	7.15	3.15
H–I	3.58	4.29
I–J	10.15	6.01
J–K	9.3	5.43
K–L	1.72	3.58
L–M	12.87	10.3
M–N	7.15	5.01
N–O	8.29	6.44

which runs along the river, starting at the base of the dam. The run ends with a small Class II rapid at the KY 7 bridge. Access is good, and navigational dangers are limited to an occasional deadfall. Runnable most of the year, the water level is dependent on releases from the dam.

Downstream of the new KY 7 bridge toward Grayson, the river flows through a wide valley, pastoral in setting but with increased human habitation. Although not nearly as scenic as the upstream sections, the river continues to make for pleasant paddling. Departing the Grayson Plain, the Little Sandy River proceeds northeast through gently rolling farmland toward the Ohio River. Increasing to 40–50 feet in width and running over a mud bottom with 9- to 16-foot mud banks, the river stays substantially the same through northern Carter County and all of Greenup County. Access is good. Navigational dangers are minimal and are once again limited primarily to deadfalls. A special point of interest in Greenup County is a historic covered bridge spanning the stream near Oldtown, off Frazer Branch Road (L). There is a fine ramp at the KY 2 bridge (N), the last access before reaching the Ohio River.

◇ **SHUTTLE** To reach the access below Grayson Lake Dam from Exit 172, keep south on KY 7. Stay with KY 7, cross Grayson Lake Dam, and turn right in the U.S. Army Corps of Engineers recreation area, toward shelter 4. The put-in is near shelter 4.

◇ **GAUGE** The USGS gauge is Little Sandy River at Grayson, KY. The minimum reading should be 150 cfs.

GPS COORDINATES

ACCESS	LATITUDE	LONGITUDE
G	N38° 15.251'	W82° 59.452'
H	N38° 17.210'	W82° 58.120'
I	N38° 17.982'	W82° 56.829'
J	N38° 21.925'	W82° 55.972'
K	N38° 24.358'	W82° 54.489'
L	N38° 25.886'	W82° 53.738'
M	N38° 29.46'	W82° 50.08'
N	N38° 31.815'	W82° 52.223'
O	N38° 34.791'	W82° 50.611'

5   TYGARTS CREEK

◇ **OVERVIEW** Originating in southwestern Carter County, Tygarts Creek flows northeast through Carter and Greenup Counties to empty into the Ohio River across the river from Portsmouth, Ohio. The best paddling section, however, runs from Olive Hill to Carter Caves State Park.

◇ **MAPS** OLIVE HILL, GRAHN, TYGARTS VALLEY (USGS)

Tygarts Creek

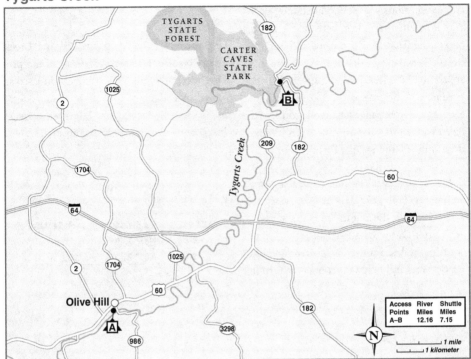

Olive Hill to
Carter Caves State Park

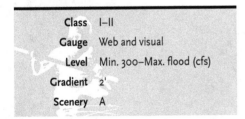

Class	I–II
Gauge	Web and visual
Level	Min. 300–Max. flood (cfs)
Gradient	2'
Scenery	A

◇ **DESCRIPTION** From Olive Hill, where the access is off Tygart Street (A) to the KY 182 bridge near Carter Caves State Resort Park (B), this creek flows through a deep, secluded gorge with evergreen- and hardwood-topped bluffs and some borderline Class II rapids. Runnable in late winter through early spring and after heavy rains, this section abounds in wildlife. Throughout the gorge, Tygarts Creek is extremely narrow (15–25 feet) and swiftly flows over a rock, sand, and gravel bottom. Navigational dangers include deadfalls, logjams, and an undercut rock on the left shortly after passing under the I-64 bridge.

From the KY 182 bridge downstream, Tygarts Creek continues to flow through a gorge for an additional 5 miles before descending into the valley south of Iron Hill. Although the beginning of this section is very scenic, the final several miles are rather lackluster (as is the remainder of the creek as it flows northeast toward the Ohio). Between Iron Hill and its mouth, Tygarts Creek can be run from November to mid-June, but it is not particularly appealing. The river's width here is 30–45 feet with steep banks of mud. Vegetation at riverside is essentially scrub weeds, and trees are conspicuously absent. Surrounding terrain is rolling farmland with some cultivation of the flattened floodplains adjoining the stream. Deadfalls and logjams are common, as are some of the less aesthetic effects of lateral erosion. One bright spot in this section, however, is a covered bridge half a mile south of the Plum Fork church in Greenup County. Access from Iron Hill to the Ohio River is poor.

◇ **SHUTTLE** The take-out boat ramp is located on Smoky Hill Lake at Carter Caves State Park. To reach the put-in from the take-out, exit Carter Caves State Park and take KY 182 South 4.7 miles. South of I-64, turn right onto US 60 West and follow it 3.5 miles to turn left onto Cross Street in Olive Hill. Go two blocks to reach Tygarts Creek and the put-in.

◇ **GAUGE** The USGS gauge, Tygarts Creek near Greenup, KY, is downstream of the preferred section of the Tygarts but can be used as an aid. A reading of 300 cfs or higher is best to float the upper section. However, a visual inspection will confirm floatability of the creek.

GPS Coordinates

ACCESS	LATITUDE	LONGITUDE
A	N38° 17.961'	W83° 10.462'
B	N38° 22.051'	W83° 6.529'

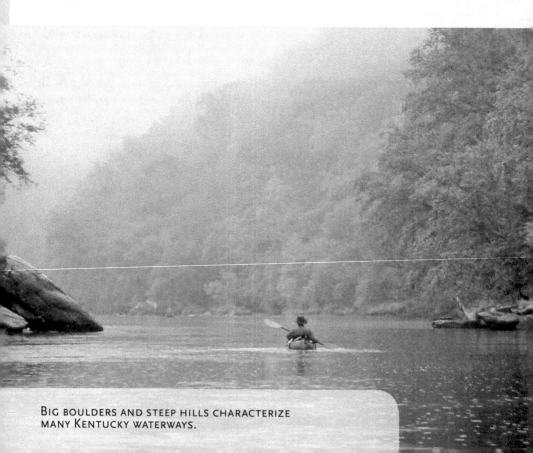

BIG BOULDERS AND STEEP HILLS CHARACTERIZE MANY KENTUCKY WATERWAYS.

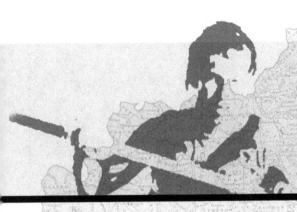

6 NORTH FORK OF THE LICKING RIVER

❖ **OVERVIEW** Flowing from east to west, the North Fork of the Licking River drains portions of Lewis, Fleming, Mason, Bracken, and Robertson Counties before joining the Middle Fork of the Licking River southeast of Falmouth. Running over a mud and limestone bottom through hilly grazing land, the North Fork often diverts around small islands of scrub vegetation.

❖ **MAPS** ORANGEBURG, MAYS LICK, SARDIS, MOUNT OLIVET, CLAYSVILLE (USGS)

Lewisburg to Riley Mill Bridge

see map on p. 30

Class	I
Gauge	Web
Level	Min. 200–Max. flood (cfs)
Gradient	2.65'
Scenery	C

❖ **DESCRIPTION** The North Fork can be canoed west of Lewisburg in Mason County November–early June but is not particularly appealing. The entire North Fork is a Class I stream with deadfalls and logjams posing the major hazards to navigation. There are numerous access points, making trips of varied lengths possible.

❖ **SHUTTLE** From Falmouth, take KY 22 East a little more than 9 miles to KY 539. Turn right onto KY 539 and follow it south 5.6 miles to Riley Mill Road. Turn right onto

North Fork of the Licking River

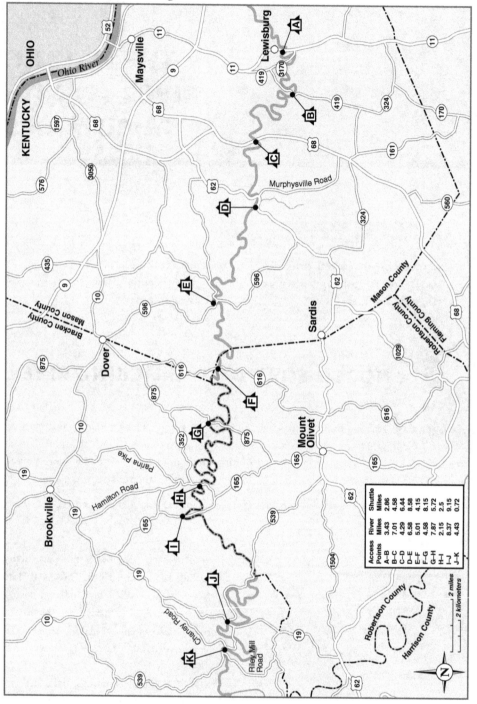

Access Points	River Miles	Shuttle Miles
A–B	3.43	2.86
B–C	7.01	4.58
C–D	4.29	6.44
D–E	6.58	8.58
E–F	5.01	4.15
F–G	4.58	8.15
G–H	7.87	5.72
H–I	2.15	2.5
I–J	8.37	9.15
J–K	4.43	0.72

Riley Mill Road and shortly reach the bridge over the North Fork Licking River and the take-out. To reach the put-in backtrack a short distance on Riley Mill Road, then turn right onto KY 539. Follow it south 10 miles, then turn left onto US 62. Follow US 62 east 10 miles, then keep straight on KY 324 East for 11 miles to reach KY 11. Turn left onto KY 11 and travel 4 miles to the bridge over the North Fork Licking.

◇ **GAUGE** The USGS gauge is North Fork Licking River at Mt. Olivet. The minimum reading should be 200 cfs.

GPS Coordinates

ACCESS	LATITUDE	LONGITUDE
A	N38° 33.228'	W83° 45.810'
B	N38° 32.961'	W83° 47.599'
C	N38° 34.199'	W83° 49.550'
D	N38° 34.162'	W83° 52.272'
E	N38° 35.488'	W83° 56.241'
F	N38° 35.411'	W83° 58.924'
G	N38° 35.698'	W84° 1.176'
H	N38° 35.971'	W84° 3.769'
I	N38° 36.553'	W84° 5.018'
J	N38° 35.027'	W84° 9.327'
K	N38° 35.090'	W84° 10.483'

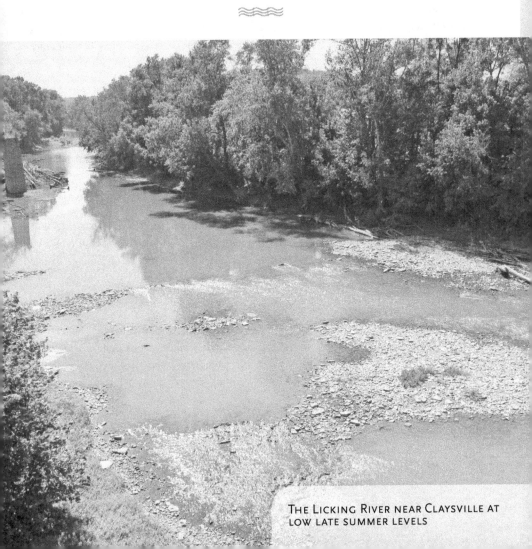

THE LICKING RIVER NEAR CLAYSVILLE AT LOW LATE SUMMER LEVELS

7 MIDDLE FORK OF THE LICKING RIVER

✧ **OVERVIEW** The Middle Fork of the Licking River originates in southern Magoffin County and flows northwest, draining portions of Morgan (where the river empties into Cave Run Lake), Menifee, Rowan, Bath, Fleming, Nicholas, Robertson, Harrison, and Pendleton Counties. From the KY 32 bridge to its confluence with the North and South Forks, the river is runnable all year long.

The Middle Fork of the Licking River runs through hilly farmland and woodlands. Flowing over a bottom of sand and mud with mud banks of varying steepness, the stream is generally lined with hardwood and scrub vegetation. Sandbars and islands of grass and scrub vegetation are common all along its length (even at relatively high water), and deadfalls are common. Many access points are on private property where permission must be obtained to put in or take out. All runs from the dam to the confluence with North Fork are Class I, but the current can be extremely swift and forceful in the spring. As it flows north, the Middle Fork broadens from 25 feet at the tailwater of the dam to 60 feet in the Blue Licks area to 95–110 feet at its confluence with the South Fork in Falmouth.

✧ **MAPS** Bangor, Salt Lick, Farmers, Colfax, Hillsboro, Sherburne, Moorefield, Cowan, Piqua, Shady Nook, Claysville, Berlin, Falmouth (USGS)

A Tailwater of Cave Run Dam to KY 32

Class	I
Gauge	Phone
Level	Min. 120–Max. flood (cfs)
Gradient	1.2'
Scenery	C+

7A **DESCRIPTION** From its origin to Cave Run Lake, the Middle Fork is littered, jammed, and generally too small to paddle. From the tailwater of the dam downstream to the KY 32 bridge near Myers, the Middle Fork is runnable from mid-October to early June, subject to water releases from the dam. It is 4 miles from the tailwater of the dam to US 60 (B), 17 miles to the KY 211 bridge (C), and 34 miles farther to KY 11 (E). The Clay Wildlife Management Area, on the west bank below KY 57 bridge, affords the opportunity for paddle camping.

✧ **SHUTTLE** From Carlisle, take KY 32 East about 7 miles to the bridge over the Middle Fork Licking River and the take-out, just after meeting KY 57 near the hamlet of Myers. To reach the put-in from the take-out, take KY 32 East 38 miles to Exit 137 on I-64. Take I-64 West 4 miles to Exit 133. From there, take KY 801 South 8 miles to turn right to cross Cave Run Lake Dam on KY 826; then turn right to the ramp at the spillway below the dam.

✧ **GAUGE** Call the U.S. Army Corps of Engineers at 606-784-9709 to receive a water release schedule from Cave Run Lake Dam. The minimum release needs to be 120 cfs.

Middle Fork of the Licking River:
Tailwater of Cave Run Dam to KY 32

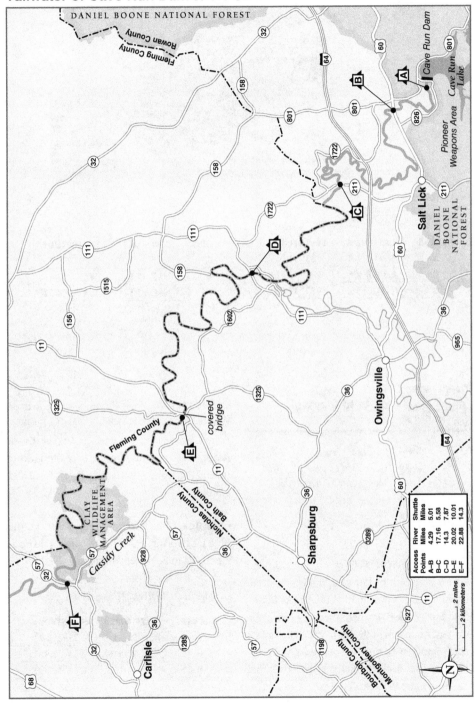

Access Points	River Miles	Shuttle Miles
A–B	4.29	5.01
B–C	17.16	5.58
C–D	14.3	7.87
D–E	20.02	10.01
E–F	22.88	14.3

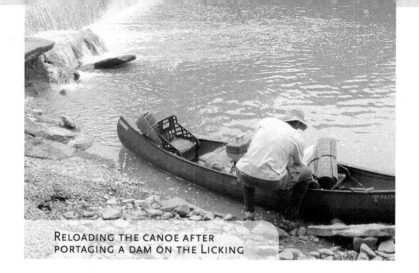

RELOADING THE CANOE AFTER
PORTAGING A DAM ON THE LICKING

GPS COORDINATES

ACCESS	LATITUDE	LONGITUDE	ACCESS	LATITUDE	LONGITUDE
A	N38° 7.049'	W83° 32.345'	D	N38° 14.113'	W83° 41.515'
B	N38° 8.406'	W83° 33.478'	E	N38° 16.846'	W83° 48.441'
C	N38° 10.565'	W83° 37.102'	F	N38° 21.544'	W83° 56.792'

B KY 32 to Claysville

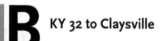

Class	I
Gauge	web
Level	Min. 150–Max. flood (cfs)
Gradient	1.1'
Scenery	C+

7B **DESCRIPTION** This section has limited access. However, paddle camping is a possibility. Paddlers can overnight at Blue Licks Battlefield State Park (G), where the river forms the western boundary of the park, which has a fine boat ramp. It is 12 miles from the KY 32 bridge down to Blue Licks Battlefield State Park and 24 more miles to Claysville (H).

✧ **SHUTTLE** To reach the upper access from Exit 121 on I-64, take KY 36 West to Carlisle. From Carlisle, take KY 32 East to Cassidy Creek Road, just before the bridge over the Licking River. Turn right onto Cassidy Creek Road and put in at the bridge over Cassidy Creek.

✧ **GAUGE** Check the Licking River at the Blue Lick Springs, KY, USGS gauge. The reading needs to be 150 cfs or higher.

GPS COORDINATES

ACCESS	LATITUDE	LONGITUDE
F	N38° 21.544'	W83° 56.792'
G	N38° 25.546'	W83° 59.922'
H	N38° 31.158'	W84° 10.990'

Middle Fork of the Licking River: KY 32 to Claysville

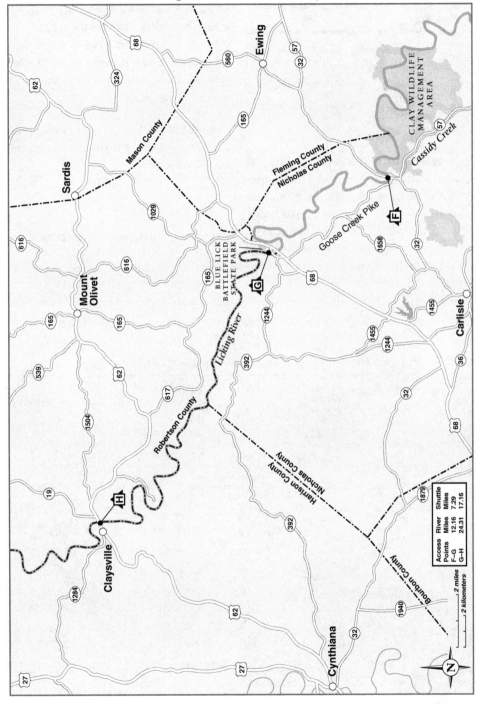

Access Points	River Miles	Shuttle Miles
F–G	12.16	7.29
G–H	24.31	17.16

C Claysville to Falmouth

Class	I
Gauge	Web
Level	Min. 120–Max. flood (cfs)
Gradient	1'
Scenery	C+

7C **DESCRIPTION** This section also has limited access. The North Fork Licking River comes in 10 miles below Claysville, substantially increasing the flow. It is 7 miles farther down to the McKenneysburg Road Bridge (I). It is 15 miles from the McKenneysburg Bridge to Falmouth (J), where a boat ramp is located on the north side of the river, off KY 22, just east of downtown Falmouth.

◆ **SHUTTLE** From the ramp and take-out on the east side of the river on KY 22 in Falmouth, take KY 22 West to US 27. Turn left onto US 27 South and travel 10 miles. Turn left onto KY 1284 and go 6.4 miles. Turn left onto US 62 to immediately reach the bridge over the Middle Fork.

◆ **GAUGE** The USGS gauge is Licking River at McKenneysburg, KY. The minimum reading should be 120 cfs.

GPS Coordinates

ACCESS	LATITUDE	LONGITUDE
H	N38° 31.158'	W84° 10.990'
I	N38° 35.875'	W84° 16.029'
J	N38° 40.611'	W84° 19.518'

Middle Fork of the Licking River: Claysville to Falmouth

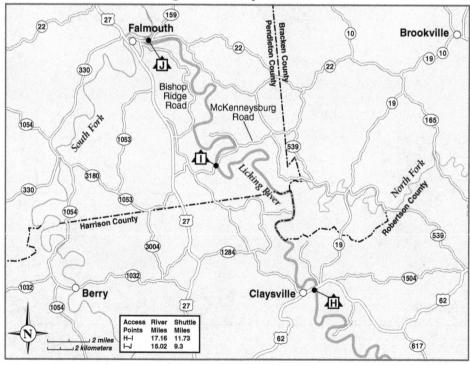

Access Points	River Miles	Shuttle Miles
H–I	17.16	11.73
I–J	15.02	9.3

8   HINKSTON CREEK

✧ **OVERVIEW** A major tributary of the South Fork of the Licking River, Hinkston Creek origi-nates in western Bath County and flows northwest along the Bourbon–Nicholas County line before joining Stoner Creek near Ruddels Mills.

✧ **MAPS** CARLISLE, MILLERSBURG, SHAWHAN (USGS)

Millersburg to Confluence with Stoner Creek

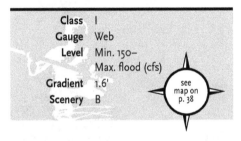

Class	I
Gauge	Web
Level	Min. 150– Max. flood (cfs)
Gradient	1.6'
Scenery	B

see map on p. 38

✧ **DESCRIPTION** Flowing over a mud and gravel bottom between 12- to 15-foot mud banks, Hinkston Creek winds through gently rolling farmland. Much of the streamside is tree lined, and several varieties of tall grasses can also be found. Runnable from Novem-ber to early June downstream of Millersburg (A), the creek is Class I with some sandbars and frequent midstream islands covered with scrub vegetation. Surrounding countryside is historically interesting with numerous stone fences, many old homes, and the Colville Covered Bridge (C). Average stream width is from 30 to 40 feet, and access is fair to good. Logjams and deadfalls are the primary haz-ards to navigation (you must put in below a 5-foot dam if starting in Millersburg). The last take-out shown on the map, Stoner Creek (E), entails a three-quarter-mile upstream paddle on Stoner Creek, so consider taking out at Ruddels Mills (D).

✧ **SHUTTLE** From Paris, take US 68 East to turn left onto KY 1940. Follow it 5.6 miles to turn left onto KY 1893 and the bridge over Stoner Creek. To reach the put-in from the take-out, take KY 1893 east 6 miles to US 68. Turn left onto US 68 East, and shortly take another left onto Shipville Road, just before the bridge over Hinkston Creek. Immediately turn right onto a dirt access on the creek.

✧ **GAUGE** The USGS gauge is Hinkston Creek near Carlisle, KY. The minimum read-ing should be 150 cfs.

GPS COORDINATES

ACCESS	LATITUDE	LONGITUDE
A	N38° 17.757'	W84° 9.104'
B	N38° 20.282'	W84° 10.212'
C	N38° 19.471'	W84° 12.186'
D	N38° 18.295'	W84° 14.283'
E	N38° 18.188'	W84° 14.977'

Hinkston Creek

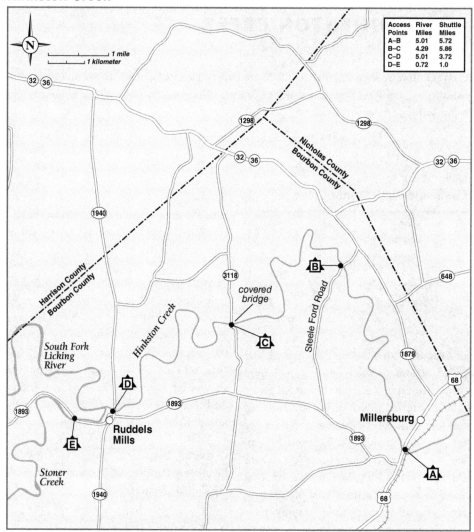

Access Points	River Miles	Shuttle Miles
A–B	5.01	5.72
B–C	4.29	5.86
C–D	5.01	3.72
D–E	0.72	1.0

9 STONER CREEK

◇ **OVERVIEW** Stoner Creek drains central Bourbon County and runs north through Paris to its confluence with Hinkston Creek. Runnable from November to mid-June north of Paris and December through April south of Paris, Stoner Creek flows through some of the world's most famous thoroughbred horse farms.

◇ **MAPS** SHAWHAN, PARIS WEST, PARIS EAST (USGS)

Stoner Creek

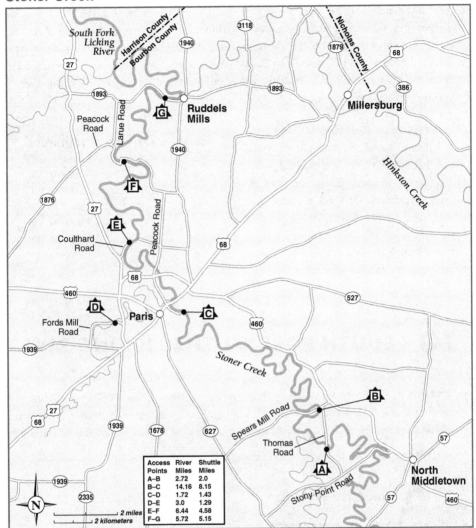

Access Points	River Miles	Shuttle Miles
A–B	2.72	2.0
B–C	14.16	8.15
C–D	1.72	1.43
D–E	3.0	1.29
E–F	6.44	4.58
F–G	5.72	5.15

Thomas Road Bridge to CR 1893 Bridge

Class	I
Gauge	Web and visual
Level	Min. 180–Max. flood (cfs)
Gradient	2.4'
Scenery	B+

◇ **DESCRIPTION** The creek itself is primarily Class I. It has numerous grass islands and flows over a mud and rock bottom between steep, 15-foot banks. Access is good north of Paris, but in the upper sections of the stream, to the south of Paris, access is difficult and often prohibited, with most put-ins and take-outs located on private property. It is here, unfortunately, that the most interesting scenery occurs. Consider paddling upstream from Paris to enjoy the scenery, then floating back. A public access is at Garrard City Park, with another off Massie Avenue. Deadfalls are the primary hazards to navigation.

✧ **SHUTTLE** From Paris, take US 68 East to turn left onto KY 1940. Follow it 5.6 miles to turn left onto KY 1893 and the bridge over Stoner Creek. To reach the put-in from the take-out, backtrack to US 68 at Paris, then take US 460 East 6.2 miles. Turn right onto Spears Mill Road and follow it 0.3 mile. Turn left onto Thomas Road and follow it 1.3 miles to the bridge over Stoner Creek.

✧ **GAUGE** Using the USGS gauge for adjacent Hinkston Creek is helpful. The USGS gauge is Hinkston Creek near Carlisle. The minimum reading should be 160 cfs. However, this method lacks precision and should be used in conjunction with a visual check of the creek.

GPS COORDINATES

ACCESS	LATITUDE	LONGITUDE
A	N38° 8.975'	W84° 9.532'
B	N38° 10.039'	W84° 9.780'
C	N38° 12.619'	W84° 14.397'
D	N38° 12.347'	W84° 16.734'
E	N38° 14.440'	W84° 16.228'
F	N38° 16.572'	W84° 16.511'
G	N38° 18.188'	W84° 14.977'

10   SOUTH FORK OF THE LICKING RIVER

✧ **OVERVIEW** The South Fork of the Licking River originates at the confluence of Hinkston and Stoner Creeks near Ruddels Mills, south of Cynthiana, and flows north over a limestone, mud, and sand bottom to join the North and Middle Forks of the Licking River near Falmouth.

✧ **MAPS** SHAWAN, CYNTHIANA, BRECKENRIDGE, BERRY, GOFORTH, FALMOUTH (USGS)

A   Ruddels Mills to Berry

Class	I
Gauge	Web
Level	Min. 3'–Max. flood
Gradient	3.4'
Scenery	B

10A DESCRIPTION Running in steep mud banks lined with silver maple and sycamore, the South Fork is Class I throughout with grass islands and numerous sandbars. The grass islands often form narrow channels that paddlers must navigate. Its average width is between 40 feet at its origin and 80–90 feet at its confluence with the other forks. A public boat ramp at point C is east of New Lair Road, on Engineer Road by the Cynthiana–Harrison County Airport. The South Fork flows through the town of Cynthiana. Access to the river is generally good. There is a public boat ramp that accesses both above and below the dam just upstream of the bridge near Robinson (E). Hazards to navigation include deadfalls as well as dams at Cynthiana, Poindexter, Robinson, and Berry (some of which exceed 5 feet in height). These must be portaged. Trips of varying lengths can be made on this river.

South Fork of the Licking River: Ruddels Mills to Berry

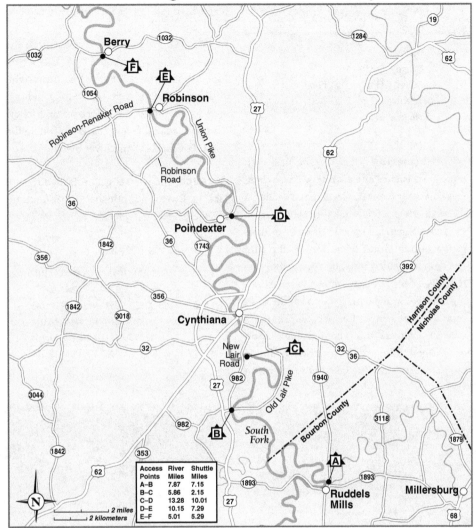

Access Points	River Miles	Shuttle Miles
A–B	7.87	7.15
B–C	5.86	2.15
C–D	13.28	10.01
D–E	10.15	7.29
E–F	5.01	5.29

◇ **SHUTTLE** From Cynthiana, take US 27 North 9 miles. Turn left onto KY 1032 and follow it 6 miles to the bridge over the South Fork in Berry. To reach the put-in from the take-out, backtrack to Cynthiana and stay south on US 27 for 7 miles. Turn left onto KY 1893 and follow it 4 miles to the bridge over Stoner Creek.

◇ **GAUGE** The USGS gauge is South Fork Licking River at Cynthiana. The minimum runnable reading is 3 feet.

GPS Coordinates

ACCESS	LATITUDE	LONGITUDE
A	N38° 18.295'	W84° 14.283'
B	N38° 20.500'	W84° 18.135'
C	N38° 22.163'	W84° 17.529'
D	N38° 26.312'	W84° 18.107'
E	N38° 29.486'	W84° 21.286'
F	N38° 31.235'	W84° 23.155'

B Berry to Falmouth

Class	I
Gauge	Web
Level	Min. 3'–Max. flood
Gradient	3.2'
Scenery	B

10B **DESCRIPTION** This section has even more grass islands and channels. These channels vary with the water level, necessitating a different route at different levels. Access to the river is generally good. Hazards to navigation include deadfalls as well as the dam at Falmouth, which must be portaged on the right. The dam at Falmouth is a popular fishing hole. Below the dam are some of the most continuous shoals on this section. Thaxton's Canoe & Paddlers' Inn (phone 859-472-2000 or visit gopaddling.com) can provide shuttle on the South Fork. The take-out in Falmouth off KY 22 (J) is actually up the Middle Fork just a bit, requiring a short upstream paddle.

SHUTTLE To reach the take-out from the intersection of US 27 and KY 22, take KY 22 East into downtown. Where KY 22 turns right, at the intersection with Main Street and just after Shelby Street, keep forward and follow the gravel road down to the Point, where the South Fork and Licking River meet.

GAUGE The USGS gauge is South Fork Licking River at Cynthiana. The minimum runnable reading is 3 feet.

GPS COORDINATES

ACCESS	LATITUDE	LONGITUDE
F	N38° 31.235'	W84° 23.155'
G	N38° 32.952'	W84° 23.742'
H	N38° 36.240'	W84° 24.011'
I	N38° 39.534'	W84° 21.204'
J	N38° 40.596'	W84° 19.515'

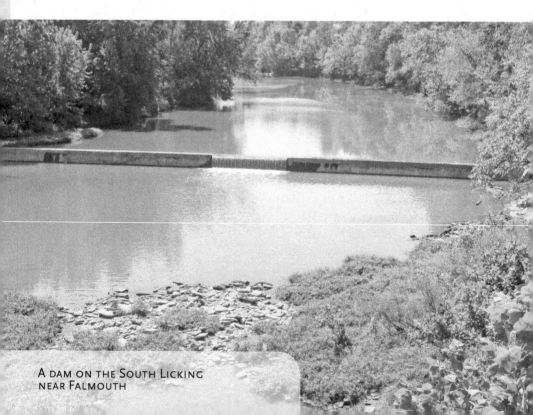

A DAM ON THE SOUTH LICKING NEAR FALMOUTH

South Fork of the Licking River: Berry to Falmouth

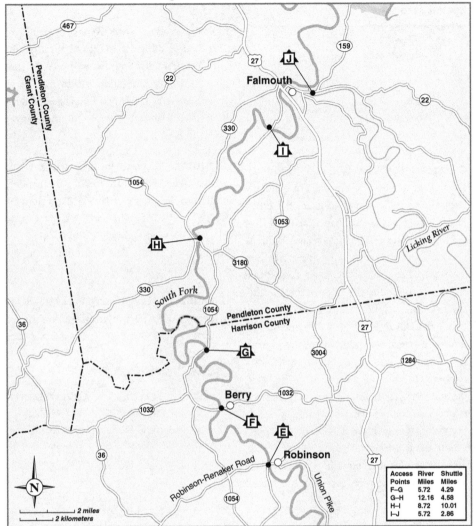

Access Points	River Miles	Shuttle Miles
F–G	5.72	4.29
G–H	12.16	4.58
H–I	8.72	10.01
I–J	5.72	2.86

11 LICKING RIVER

◇ **OVERVIEW** The Licking River below the confluence of its three forks is a big river and is runnable all year. Its scenery is pleasant, with the river winding in lengthy curves through broad valleys bordered by tall hills and ridges.

◇ **MAPS** FALMOUTH, BUTLER, DeMOSSVILLE, ALEXANDRIA, NEWPORT, COVINGTON (USGS)

Falmouth to Locust Pike Park

Class	I
Gauge	Web
Level	Min. 120–
	Max. flood (cfs)
Gradient	1.2'
Scenery	C+

⟡ DESCRIPTION The banks of the Main Licking, as it is locally known, are generally steep on one side and sloping on the other. Flat terraces occur frequently about 5 feet up from the waterline. Its average width is 190–220 feet. Trees, mostly hardwoods, line the banks. For a large, navigable river, there is a conspicuous absence of powerboat traffic, due to shoals and the scarcity of access points. Below the US 27 bridge (B) through Kenton County north to Newport, where the Licking River empties into the Ohio River, the railroad effectively monopolizes the west bank. Beyond the sprawling switchyards, steep ridges make it almost impossible to reach the water. Along the east bank in Campbell County, large farms and other types of private property buffer the stream. Comparatively long distances between access points, then,

limit this section's attractiveness to paddlers. The level of difficulty is Class I throughout, and occasional floating debris represents the only hazard to navigation. Access, as mentioned, is scarce but is reasonably good where it exists. Thaxton's Canoe Rental operates on US 27 in Butler.

⟡ SHUTTLE To reach the Locust Pike Park access, take US 27 North to KY 536. Turn left on KY 536 West to reach KY 177. Turn right on KY 177 North and follow it to KY 1930. Turn right on KY 1930 and follow it to Locust Pike. Turn left on Locust Pike and follow it to the boat ramp on the right.

⟡ GAUGE The USGS gauge is Licking River at Catawba, KY. The minimum reading should be 120.

GPS COORDINATES

ACCESS	LATITUDE	LONGITUDE
A	N38° 40.616'	W84° 19.505'
B	N38° 47.366'	W84° 22.046'
C	N38° 55.215'	W84° 26.779'
D	N38° 58.090'	W84° 27.841'

Licking River: Falmouth to Locust Pike Park

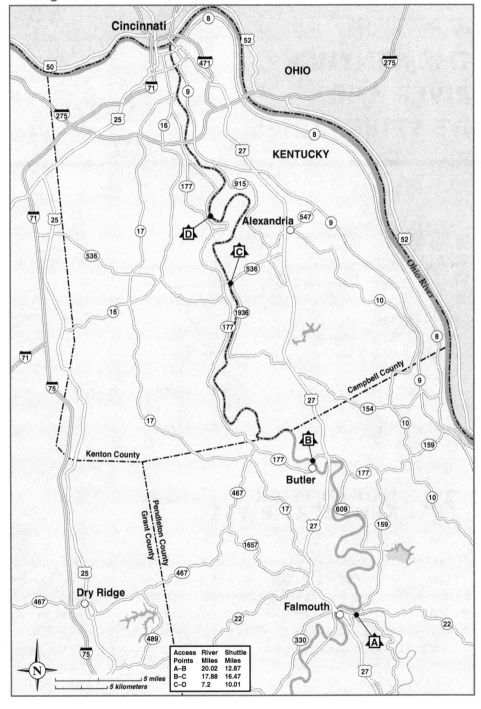

Access Points	River Miles	Shuttle Miles
A–B	20.02	12.87
B–C	17.88	16.47
C–D	7.2	10.01

PART THREE
THE KENTUCKY RIVER AND ITS TRIBUTARIES

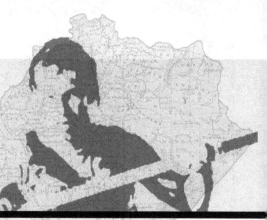

12 NORTH FORK OF THE KENTUCKY RIVER

◊ **OVERVIEW** The North Fork of the Kentucky River originates in the mountains of southeastern Kentucky near Whitesburg and flows northwest, draining the counties of Letcher, Perry, Breathitt, and Lee. There are 140 paddleable miles before the North Fork meets the South Fork and Middle Fork in Beattyville. This is a bona fide mountainous coal country, where the only flat land is directly along any watercourse slicing through the hills. The North Fork is no exception, and much of the streamside is settled or farmed. The North Fork is runnable in its upper reaches (Roxana to Viper) during the winter and early spring only. Downstream, from Viper to Jackson, the river can be paddled from late October to mid-June. Below Jackson, the North Fork of the Kentucky is usually runnable all year.

◊ **MAPS** Roxana, Blackey, Vicco, Hazard South, Hazard North, Krypton, Haddix, Quicksand, Jackson, Tallega, Campton, Zachariah, Beattyville (USGS)

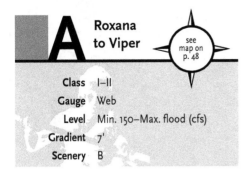

A Roxana to Viper

see map on p. 48

Class	I–II
Gauge	Web
Level	Min. 150–Max. flood (cfs)
Gradient	7'
Scenery	B

12A **DESCRIPTION** In the upper sections, the river is 35–40 feet wide and flows over a mud and gravel bed through steep, wooded valleys and coal country. As Line Fork enters the stream at the Perry–Letcher County line, water volume increases significantly, and the river widens to approximately 55–60 feet. Although the terrain is rugged, humans and their habitat are visible all along the upper North Fork. Trees overhang the stream in the extreme upper section (above Blackey [B]) but give way to thick scrub vegetation further downstream. There's a boat ramp in Ulvah (C). Paddling is interesting, with numerous small shoals and rapids (Class I+). Deadfalls pose the only major peril to navigation.

SHUTTLE To reach the take-out from Hazard, take KY 15 South/KY 7 North 8 miles to the bridge over Maces Creek, just before it merges into the North Fork. To reach the put-in from the take-out, take KY 7 North 18 miles. Turn right onto KY 2036 and follow it 4 miles to the put-in on your right at the bridge over Mill Branch at its confluence with North Fork.

GAUGE The USGS gauge is North Fork Kentucky River at Whitesburg. The minimum reading should be 150 cfs.

GPS COORDINATES

ACCESS	LATITUDE	LONGITUDE
A	N37° 6.543'	W82° 56.999'
B	N37° 8.313'	W82° 59.342'
C	N37° 7.709'	W83° 3.106'
D	N37° 8.029'	W83° 4.622'
E	N37° 10.400'	W83° 5.498'
F	N37° 10.985'	W83° 8.944'

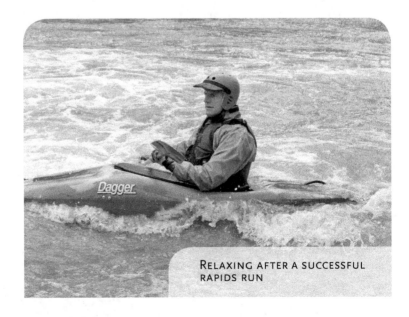

RELAXING AFTER A SUCCESSFUL RAPIDS RUN

North Fork of the Kentucky River: Roxana to Viper

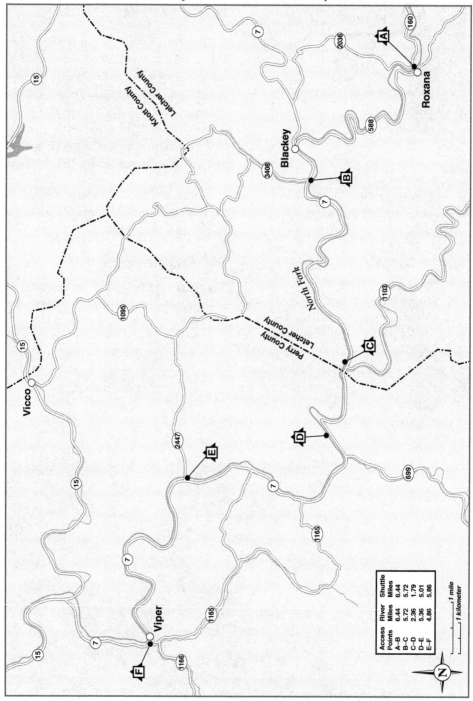

Access Points	River Miles	Shuttle Miles
A–B	6.44	6.44
B–C	5.72	5.72
C–D	2.36	1.79
D–E	5.36	5.01
E–F	4.86	5.86

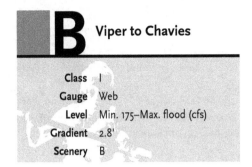

B Viper to Chavies

Class	I
Gauge	Web
Level	Min. 175–Max. flood (cfs)
Gradient	2.8'
Scenery	B

12B DESCRIPTION This section of the North Fork passes through the growing town of Hazard (H), where you can access the river near Triangle Park. Downstream of Hazard, paddlers can enjoy the ramp at Neace Gorman Park (I). The gradient is less than the upper section, but shoals keep you moving along. Though detracting from the wilderness atmosphere, the small towns, frame

North Fork of the Kentucky River: Viper to Chavies

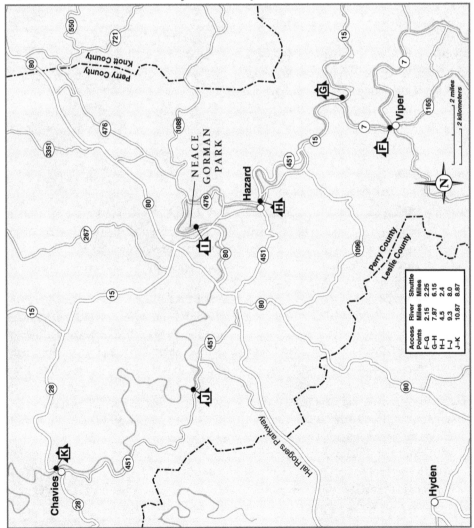

Access Points	River Miles	Shuttle Miles
F–G	2.15	2.25
G–H	7.87	6.15
H–I	4.5	2.4
I–J	9.3	8.0
J–K	10.87	8.87

houses, wooden footbridges, and porch-front rockers present an enduring and picturesque perspective of eastern Kentucky mountain living. The river itself is winding and has steep banks that make access generally difficult, even at bridges. Difficulty notwithstanding, additional access points along the section make trips of varied distances possible. Much of the river can be scouted from KY 15 south of Hazard. As KY 15 intersects the river south of Hazard, the North Fork sinks into increasingly deep banks. Even with a highway on the west and a railroad on the east, access is difficult. Scenery, however, remains beautiful.

✧ **SHUTTLE** To reach the take-out from Hazard, follow KY 15 South 15 miles to the bridge over the North Fork in Chavies. To reach the put-in from the take-out, backtrack to Hazard on KY 15 and follow it 5 miles. Then join KY 7 North and follow it 2 miles to the bridge over Maces Creek at its confluence with North Fork.

✧ **GAUGE** The USGS gauge is North Fork Kentucky River at Whitesburg. The minimum reading should be 175 cfs.

GPS COORDINATES

ACCESS	LATITUDE	LONGITUDE
F	N37° 10.985'	W83° 8.944'
G	N37° 12.379'	W83° 7.902'
H	N37° 14.803'	W83° 11.660'
I	N37° 14.803'	W83° 11.660'
J	N37° 16.784'	W83° 18.347'
K	N37° 20.875'	W83° 21.189'

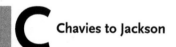

C   Chavies to Jackson

Class	I
Gauge	Web
Level	Min. 175–Max. flood (cfs)
Gradient	2.7'
Scenery	B–

12C **DESCRIPTION** Signs of human habitation are more frequent and the scenery far less picturesque than farther upstream. The river valley broadens here, and farm fields become more common. Rapids and shoals disappear as the stream settles into mud banks. Access is somewhat limited the first 17 miles below Chavies; however, after that, access can be had in Copeland at the old low-water bridge off KY 1110 (M), off KY 15 where a bridge crosses over to Quicksand (N), and in Jackson at Douthitt Park. A big bend of the river was cut off in Jackson, to prevent flooding and there is now a rapid where the bend was short-cutted.

✧ **SHUTTLE** The take-out is at Douthitt Park, off North Point Avenue in Jackson. To reach the put-in from the take-out, take North Point Avenue a short distance to KY 30. Turn right onto KY 30 and follow it east 3.5 miles. Keep straight to join KY 15 South and follow it 19 miles. Turn right onto KY 28 West and follow it 5.8 miles to the bridge over the North Fork near Chavies.

✧ **GAUGE** The USGS gauge is North Fork Kentucky River at Whitesburg. The minimum reading should be 175 cfs.

North Fork of the Kentucky River: Chavies to Jackson

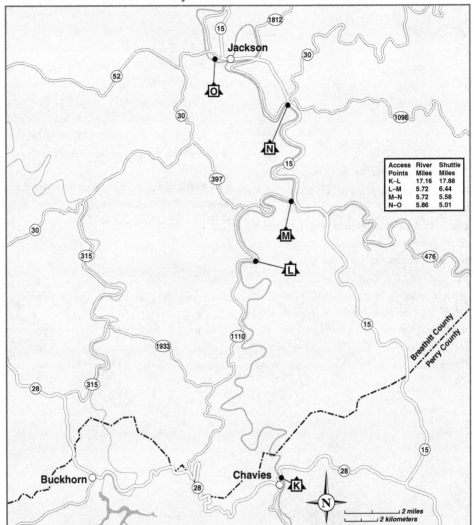

Access Points	River Miles	Shuttle Miles
K–L	17.16	17.88
L–M	5.72	6.44
M–N	5.72	5.58
N–O	5.86	5.01

ACCESS	LATITUDE	LONGITUDE	ACCESS	LATITUDE	LONGITUDE
K	N37° 20.875'	W83° 21.189'	N	N37° 32.057'	W83° 20.879'
L	N37° 27.347'	W83° 22.152'	O	N37° 33.407'	W83° 23.724'
M	N37° 32.064'	W83° 20.877'			

D Jackson to Beattyville

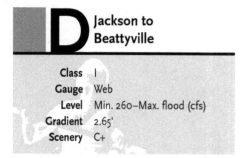

Class	I
Gauge	Web
Level	Min. 260–Max. flood (cfs)
Gradient	2.65'
Scenery	C+

12D **DESCRIPTION** As the North Fork flows north through Jackson toward Beattyville, the surrounding hills (known locally as mountains) become smaller and the river widens to an average of 80 feet and expands to 110 feet at its confluence with the Middle Fork of the Kentucky. Though runnable all year, this section lacks the intimacy and beauty typical of the upper sections. Alternative access points include the KY 541 bridge where there is a ramp (P) and the KY 2016 bridge (Q). Between these two bridges is a 30-mile stretch with no public access.

◇ **SHUTTLE** The take-out in Beattyville is located just west of the KY 52 bridge over the North Fork. Look left just on the west side of the bridge for River Road. Turn left here and look left for a small public park next to the Beattyville City Hall, an old house. To reach the put-in from the take-out, take KY 52 East 21.4 miles. Turn left onto KY 30 East and follow it 1.6 miles. Turn right onto North Point Avenue and reach the ramp at Douthitt Park.

◇ **GAUGE** The USGS gauge is North Fork Kentucky River at Whitesburg. The minimum reading should be 260 cfs.

GPS Coordinates

ACCESS	LATITUDE	LONGITUDE
O	N37° 33.407'	W83° 23.724'
P	N37° 36.098'	W83° 26.867'
Q	N37° 36.144'	W83° 38.508'
R	N37° 34.187'	W83° 42.481'

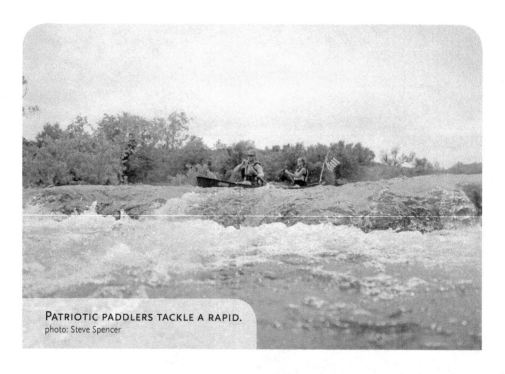

PATRIOTIC PADDLERS TACKLE A RAPID.
photo: Steve Spencer

North Fork of the Kentucky River: Jackson to Beattyville

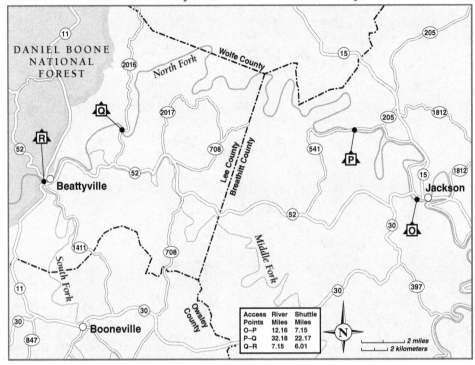

Access Points	River Miles	Shuttle Miles
O–P	12.16	7.15
P–Q	32.18	22.17
Q–R	7.15	6.01

13 MIDDLE FORK OF THE KENTUCKY RIVER

◇ **OVERVIEW** The Middle Fork of the Kentucky River originates in the southeastern Kentucky mountains of Leslie County and flows north through the tip of Perry County into Buckhorn Lake, and from there north through Breathitt County into Lee County, where it joins the North Fork of the Kentucky near Beattyville.

◇ **MAPS** HOSKINSTON, CUTSHIN, HYDEN EAST, HYDEN WEST, BUCKHORN CANOE, COWCREEK, TALLEGA, BEATTYVILLE (USGS); DANIEL BOONE NATIONAL FOREST, CENTRAL SECTION

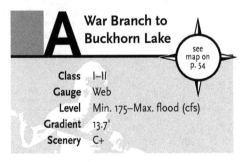

A War Branch to Buckhorn Lake

see map on p. 54

Class	I–II
Gauge	Web
Level	Min. 175–Max. flood (cfs)
Gradient	13.7'
Scenery	C+

13A **DESCRIPTION** The upper waters of the Middle Fork roll out of the hills in the western portion of Leslie County in the Daniel Boone National Forest. Although the upper reaches are crowded with small mountain communities, the river valley and surrounding hills are nevertheless extremely beautiful.

Middle Fork of the Kentucky River: War Branch to Buckhorn Lake

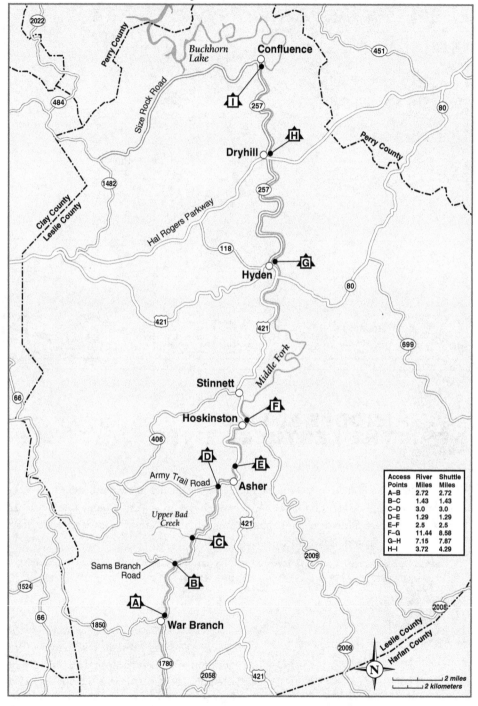

Access Points table:

Access Points	River Miles	Shuttle Miles
A–B	2.72	2.72
B–C	1.43	1.43
C–D	3.0	3.0
D–E	1.29	1.29
E–F	2.5	2.5
F–G	11.44	8.58
G–H	7.15	7.87
H–I	3.72	4.29

The river flows over a rock and gravel bed with almost continuous Class I+ and Class II rapids and shoals. Runnable in late winter and early spring, the upper section is paralleled by KY 1780, from which the run can be scouted. Hazards, including deadfalls, low bridges, and concrete fords, are easily spotted. The river is small, averaging 25–35 feet in width. Banks are 6–10 feet in height and easily traversed; access is good. The riverside of the banks is well vegetated, but most trees are situated somewhat back on the floodplain away from the river, providing the mixed blessing of being able to see both the human habitation and the truly spectacular surrounding hills ("mountains") as you paddle along.

Near the intersection of KY 1780 and US 421, the river collects several major tributaries and proceeds to follow US 421 north toward Hyden. This section is also characterized by extremely mild whitewater (Class I+), but it is of a more intermittent nature. Access once again is good, and the scenery is much improved as the river moves away from the line of houses and barns that dot the headwaters. Runnable from late November to early June, this section passes through beautiful wilderness hill terrain before emerging in Hoskinston (F). Beyond Hoskinston and Stinnett, the river again slips into the forest to rejoin civilization in Hyden (G). Occasional deadfalls and a 5-foot dam as the river approaches the Leslie County High School complex south of Hyden are the only dangers to navigation.

At Hyden, where this is a fine access at City Park, the river averages 50 feet in width and has descended into a luxurious green valley sprinkled with cabins on the hills overlooking the river. Its banks are mud and are extremely tall and steep. Above the steep banks, a gorge rises with exposed rock visible. This can best be appreciated during the colder months when the foliage of trees along the banks does not obstruct the view. From Hyden to Buckhorn Lake, the river smooths considerably and has only a few riffles and small waves. Access is good where it is available, including Confluence Recreation Area (I). This section is normally runnable from November to early June. Trace Branch Recreation Area on Buckhorn Lake, which has camping, is just down the lake from Confluence Recreation Area.

⟡ SHUTTLE To reach the take-out from Hyden, take KY 257 North 11.1 miles to the Confluence Recreation Area and boat ramp. To reach the put-in from the take-out, backtrack on KY 257 to Hyden and take US 421 South 11.3 miles. Turn right onto KY 1780 and follow it 7 miles. Turn right onto KY 1850 and immediately drop to the bridge over the Middle Fork at War Branch.

⟡ GAUGE The USGS gauge is Middle Fork Kentucky River at Tallega. The minimum reading should be 175 cfs.

GPS COORDINATES

ACCESS	LATITUDE	LONGITUDE
A	N36° 58.298'	W83° 26.946'
B	N36° 59.992'	W83° 26.569'
C	N37° 0.851'	W83° 25.848'
D	N37° 2.523'	W83° 24.768'
E	N37° 3.146'	W83° 24.031'
F	N37° 4.681'	W83° 23.534'
G	N37° 9.822'	W83° 22.369'
H	N37° 13.370'	W83° 22.599'
I	N37° 16.208'	W83° 22.975'

B Buckhorn Dam to Beattyville

Class	I
Gauge	Web
Level	Min. 210–Max. flood (cfs)
Gradient	1.7'
Scenery	C+

13B **DESCRIPTION** From the tailwaters of the Buckhorn Dam to the mouth of Turkey Creek in Breathitt County, the river widens somewhat but otherwise remains essentially the same. Habitation along the Middle Fork increases sharply along this section as the river departs the national forest. This section is runnable almost all year, and access is good. The shuttle route follows the river almost the entire way and makes trips of varied lengths easy.

From the mouth of Turkey Creek (near Guerrant) to the Lee County line, the Middle Fork flows through hilly woods and farm country, but population is sparse, and fewer dwellings are visible from the river. Between Turkey Creek and its confluence with the North Fork of the Kentucky, the Middle Fork swells to 110–130 feet in width. Like the North Fork, the Middle Fork in Lee County lacks the dramatic scenery and continually changing vistas of the upper sections.

◊ **SHUTTLE** The take-out is on River Drive, just west of the KY 11 bridge over the North Fork Kentucky River in Beattyville, just above its confluence with the Middle Fork. To reach the put-in from the take-out, follow KY 11 South 9.6 miles to Booneville. In Booneville, keep straight, joining KY 28 East for 17.7 miles to reach Buckhorn. In Buckhorn, stay straight, joining KY 1387 for 0.3 mile, then veer left onto Campground Road; stay right to reach the boat ramp at the tailwater below Buckhorn Dam.

◊ **GAUGE** The USGS gauge is Middle Fork Kentucky River at Tallega. The minimum reading should be 210 cfs.

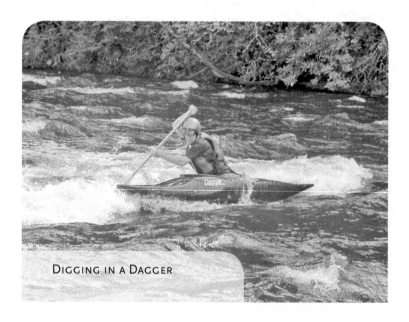

DIGGING IN A DAGGER

Middle Fork of the Kentucky River: Buckhorn Dam to Beattyville

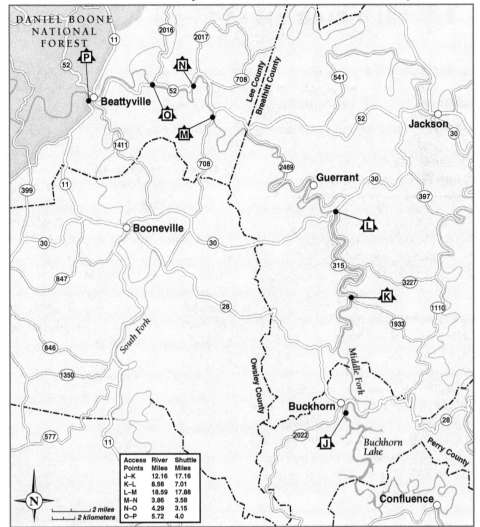

Access Points	River Miles	Shuttle Miles
J–K	12.16	17.16
K–L	8.58	7.01
L–M	18.59	17.88
M–N	3.86	3.58
N–O	4.29	3.15
O–P	5.72	4.0

GPS Coordinates

ACCESS	LATITUDE	LONGITUDE
J	N37° 20.448'	W83° 28.232'
K	N37° 25.381'	W83° 27.956'
L	N37° 29.246'	W83° 28.791'
M	N37° 33.311'	W83° 35.657'

ACCESS	LATITUDE	LONGITUDE
N	N37° 34.649'	W83° 36.762'
O	N37° 34.649'	W83° 36.762'
P	N37° 34.187'	W83° 42.481'

14 RED BIRD RIVER

◇ **OVERVIEW** The Red Bird River is the main tributary of the South Fork of the Kentucky River. Running over a bed of rock, gravel, and mud, the Red Bird winds through the Daniel Boone National Forest, draining the eastern half of Clay County.

◇ **MAPS** CREEKVILLE, BIG CREEK (USGS); DANIEL BOONE NATIONAL FOREST, CENTRAL SECTION

Queensdale to South Fork Kentucky River

Class	I+
Gauge	Visual
Level	Min. 180–Max. flood (cfs)
Gradient	7.2'
Scenery	B

◇ **DESCRIPTION** Runnable in late fall and spring, the river can best be described as a busy Class I with almost continuous riffles, small waves, and shoals. At higher water, several of the shoals and small rapids may be classified as borderline Class II. The Red Bird valley is one of the most beautiful in the Daniel Boone National Forest, with steep hills looming above the river and lush vegetation everywhere. Some human habitation is in evidence along the Red Bird River, but it does not usually detract from the beauty of the stream. Banks are 5–8 feet high and of varying steepness. Access is good a little below from the Red Bird Hospital (A) to the KY 80 bridge (F), as roads parallel the Red Bird the whole way. This allows for scouting and trips of varied lengths. Average width is 30–40 feet throughout, and concrete fords and deadfalls represent the only navigational hazards.

◇ **SHUTTLE** To reach the take-out from Manchester, take US 421 South for a mile to KY 80 East/Hal Rogers Parkway and follow it 13.5 miles. Turn left onto KY 66 North and travel 2 miles. Turn left onto Eriline Road and quickly reach the bridge over the Red Bird River. To reach the put-in from the take-out, return to KY 66, turn right (south), and follow KY 66 for 19.6 miles to the bridge over Phillips Fork, just before intersecting KY 1850/Phillips Fork Road.

◇ **GAUGE** Nearly the entire river can be scouted by parallel roads. The Red Bird should be runnable when the South Fork Kentucky is a little high.

GPS COORDINATES

ACCESS	LATITUDE	LONGITUDE
A	N37° 1.249'	W83° 32.027'
B	N37° 2.141'	W83° 31.965'
C	N37° 4.410'	W83° 32.480'
D	N37° 5.810'	W83° 33.427'
E	N37° 6.991'	W83° 33.843'
F	N37° 9.818'	W83° 35.000'
G	N37° 11.476'	W83° 35.727'

Red Bird River

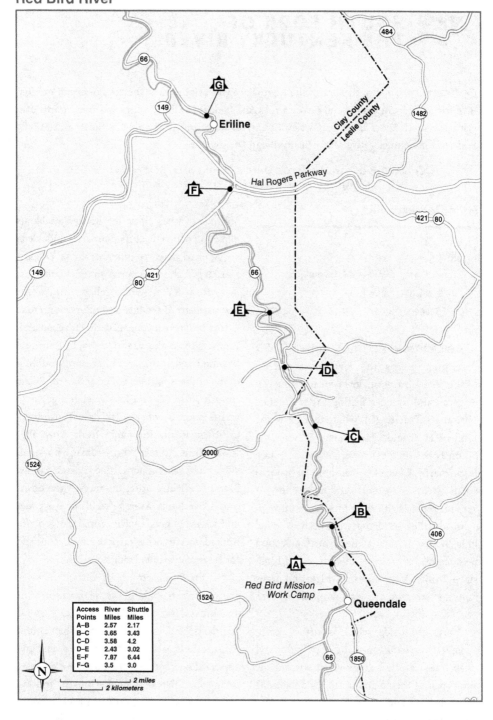

Access Points	River Miles	Shuttle Miles
A–B	2.57	2.17
B–C	3.65	3.43
C–D	3.58	4.2
D–E	2.43	3.02
E–F	7.87	6.44
F–G	3.5	3.0

15 SOUTH FORK OF THE KENTUCKY RIVER

✧ **OVERVIEW** The South Fork of the Kentucky River originates at the confluence of the Red Bird River, Bullskin Creek, and Goose Creek (at Oneida) in Clay County and flows north over primarily mud banks through Owsley County to its confluence with the North and Middle Forks of the Kentucky River, near Beattyville in Lee County.

✧ **MAPS** Big Tree, Mistletoe, Oneida, Booneville, Beattyville (USGS); Daniel Boone National Forest, Central Section

Eriline to Beattyville

Class	I (II)
Gauge	Web
Level	Min. 225–Max. flood (cfs)
Gradient	3.3'
Scenery	B

✧ **DESCRIPTION** The first part of this description traces the lowermost reaches of the Red Bird as it flows north from Hal Rogers Parkway near Eriline (A) to Oneida. Forming at Oneida (C), where there is a fine ramp near Oneida Elementary School, the South Fork averages 35–50 feet in width and is primarily Class I with some occasional small shoals. The surrounding scenery is very pleasant as the river meanders through a broad valley bordered with high, wooded hills. Access is fair (at best) in this section because of a scarcity of crossings and high, steep banks. Vegetation is thick and trees line the streamside. Navigational hazards consist mainly of deadfalls.

North of Oneida (which is further downstream), the banks remain very high and steep. Trees are less frequent at streamside, and much of the surrounding floodplain has been terraced and farmed. The river is less scenic here than upstream, but the general absence of trees along the immediate banks allows a good view of the bordering hillsides.

Approximately 3 miles north of Oneida, near Teges, the river turns sharply to the east away from KY 11 (which follows the stream downstream of Oneida and offers numerous access points) into dense, secluded woodland. From here to the Clay–Owsley County line lies the most scenic and interesting paddling of the entire South Fork. The access off Rocky Branch Road (E) is a low-water bridge, as is access point G, where Wolf Creek Road links to River Road. Runnable from November to mid-June, this section is alive with small shoals and several borderline Class II rapids. Sloping hillsides bring the forest right down to the riverbank. Average width is 45–55 feet and access is good. Navigational dangers are limited to an occasional deadfall, concrete fords, and low-water bridges.

As the South Fork flows through Owsley County, leaving behind the national forest, it encounters broader valleys, scenic, pastoral farmland, and increased human habitation. Riffles and shoals are infrequent here and disappear altogether after the South Fork passes Booneville. Between Booneville (I) and its confluence with the North and Middle Forks (K), the South Fork averages 70–90 feet in

South Fork of the Kentucky River

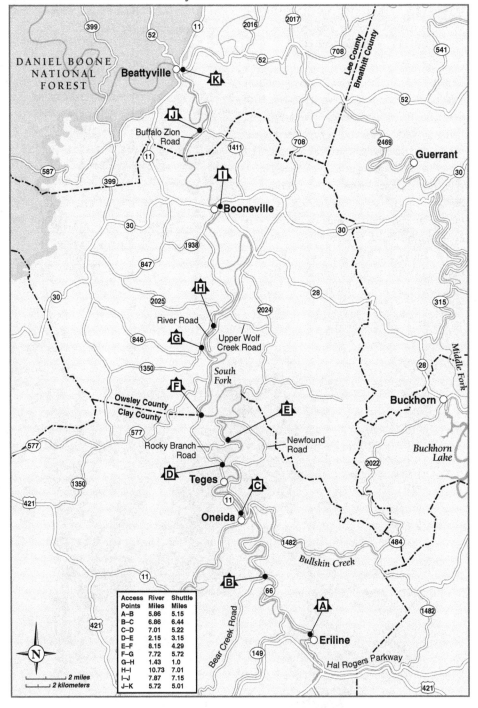

DANIEL BOONE NATIONAL FOREST

Beattyville

Buffalo Zion Road

Booneville

Guerrant

River Road

Upper Wolf Creek Road

South Fork

Owsley County

Clay County

Rocky Branch Road

Newfound Road

Buckhorn

Buckhorn Lake

Middle Fork

Teges

Oneida

Bullskin Creek

Eriline

Bear Creek Road

Hal Rogers Parkway

Lee County

Breathitt County

Access Points	River Miles	Shuttle Miles
A–B	5.86	5.15
B–C	6.86	6.44
C–D	7.01	5.22
D–E	2.15	3.15
E–F	8.15	4.29
F–G	7.72	5.72
G–H	1.43	1.0
H–I	10.73	7.01
I–J	7.87	7.15
J–K	5.72	5.01

N

2 miles
2 kilometers

width and is runnable all year. Access is fair to good. It is 13 miles from Eriline to Oneida, 36 miles from Oneida to Booneville, and 14 miles from Booneville to Beattyville.

◇ **SHUTTLE** The access in Beattyville is just west of the KY 52 bridge over the North Fork Kentucky River. Turn onto River Drive and follow it just a few feet to a park on the left, beside the Beattyville City Hall offices. You have to paddle upstream on the North Fork a very short distance below the KY 11 bridge on the South Fork to reach this access. To reach the put-in from the take-out, stay with KY 11 South for 30 miles to turn left onto KY 66 South. Follow KY 66 South 11.3 miles, then turn right onto Eriline Road and reach the bridge over the Red Bird River.

◇ **GAUGE** The USGS gauge is South Fork Kentucky River at Booneville. The minimum reading should be 225 cfs.

GPS Coordinates

ACCESS	LATITUDE	LONGITUDE
A	N37° 11.520'	W83° 35.645'
B	N37° 13.733'	W83° 37.916'
C	N37° 16.307'	W83° 39.184'
D	N37° 18.250'	W83° 40.171'
E	N37° 19.251'	W83° 39.863'
F	N37° 20.257'	W83° 41.281'
G	N37° 22.984'	W83° 41.258'
H	N37° 23.789'	W83° 40.613'
I	N37° 28.514'	W83° 40.251'
J	N37° 31.708'	W83° 41.322'
K	N37° 34.187'	W83° 42.481'

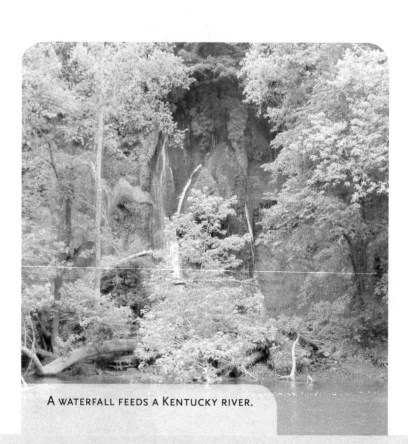

A WATERFALL FEEDS A KENTUCKY RIVER.

16 KENTUCKY RIVER BELOW THE FORKS

◇ **OVERVIEW** The Kentucky River from Beattyville to Frankfort would be a better paddling stream were it not for the abundance of powerboats, both pleasure and commercial. The Kentucky River is scenic, running first through forested hills and well-kept farmland, later curving beneath 400-foot exposed rock palisades, and finally emerging into a broad, fertile plain bordered by tall, wooded ridges. Access is plentiful and usually good. Dangers to navigation include ten dams (exclusive of No. 4 below Frankfort), floating debris, and of course, the ever-present armada of power craft. A Class I river, the Kentucky is runnable all year. Its banks are mud and usually steep. Numerous trip possibilities exist along this stretch. Highlights include historic Camp Nelson downstream of Lock 8, High Bridge and the mouth of the Dix River below Dix Dam (Herrington Lake) just upstream of Lock 7, and the City of Frankfort (the capital of Kentucky) above Lock 4.

Visitors are welcome at all of the locks, and the lock grounds are suitable for picnicking, putting in, or taking out. Two locks (10 and 8) have beaches adjoining them. You can usually leave shuttle vehicles parked at the locks while you are running the river, but be sure to check with the lockmaster to find out what time the grounds are closed. Be aware that locks 5, 6, 7, 8, 9, 10, 11, 12, 13, and 14 have been closed until further notice. Locks 1–4 are open during summer boating season but check the Kentucky River Authority's website for the latest on the locks at finance.ky.gov/offices/kra.

When approaching the locks from the river, all must obviously be portaged. If you are in a large group or arrive at the lock at the same time as a powerboat, the lockmaster will normally allow you to lock through. Though not as fast as carrying around, locking through is fun and interesting, particularly if there are children in the group.

◇ **MAPS** NEW LIBERTY, WORTHVILLE, VEVAY SOUTH, CARROLLTON, FRANKFORT EAST, FRANKFORT WEST, POLSGROVE, SWITZER, GRATZ, SALVISA, TYRONE, VALLEY VIEW, LITTLE HICKMAN, BUCKEYE, WILMORE, HARRODSBURG, PANOLA, PALMER, UNION CITY, WINCHESTER, FORD, RICHMOND NORTH, VALLEY VIEW (USGS)

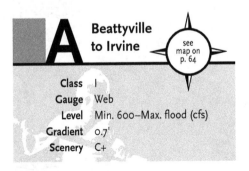

A Beattyville to Irvine

see map on p. 64

Class	I
Gauge	Web
Level	Min. 600–Max. flood (cfs)
Gradient	0.7'
Scenery	C+

16A DESCRIPTION The forks of the Kentucky River gather at Beattyville to form the Kentucky, averaging 80–105 feet wide here. This upper stretch is in coal country. A railroad parallels the river its entire length. The lower stretch has the advantage of boat ramps at the landings. Lock 14 is encountered 3 miles below Beattyville. The KY 399 bridge is 4 miles farther. Lock 13 is 10 miles below KY 399. It is 21 miles between Lock 13 and Lock 12, and 4 more miles to Irvine.

Kentucky River Below the Forks: Beattyville to Irvine

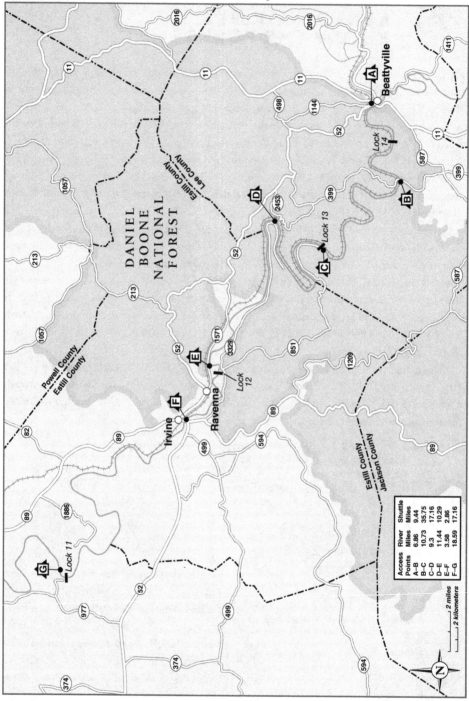

Access Points	River Miles	Shuttle Miles
A–B	6.86	9.44
B–C	10.73	35.75
C–D	9.3	17.16
D–E	11.44	10.29
E–F	3.58	2.86
F–G	18.59	17.16

✧ **SHUTTLE** The take-out is on the southwest side of the KY 52 bridge over the Kentucky River in Irvine. To reach the put-in from the take-out, take KY 52 east out of Irvine and follow it 24 miles to Beattyville. Turn right on River Drive to reach an access on your right.

✧ **GAUGE** The USGS gauge is Kentucky River at Lock 14/Heidelberg. The minimum reading should be 600 cfs.

GPS COORDINATES

ACCESS	LATITUDE	LONGITUDE
A	N37° 34.187'	W83° 42.481'
B	N37° 32.996'	W83° 46.413'
C	N37° 36.177'	W83° 49.869'
D	N37° 38.206'	W83° 48.423'
E	N37° 40.914'	W83° 55.799'
F	N37° 41.836'	W83° 58.536'
G	N37° 47.052'	W84° 6.153'

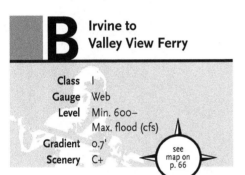

B Irvine to Valley View Ferry

Class	I
Gauge	Web
Level	Min. 600–
	Max. flood (cfs)
Gradient	0.7'
Scenery	C+

see map on p. 66

16B **DESCRIPTION** Points of interest include Fort Boonesborough State Park (with beach and campground) just below Lock 10 (K), and a 30-foot waterfall one-half mile up Boone Creek (entering the Kentucky River on the right just upstream of the I-75 bridge). The river averages 95–125 feet wide on this stretch. It is 18.5 miles from Irvine to Lock 11. The Red River comes in 10 miles below Lock 11. It is 16.5 miles to Fort Boonesborough State Park and Lock 10 from the Red River (H), and 20.5 miles farther to Valley View Ferry (N) from the park.

✧ **SHUTTLE** To reach the take-out from Richmond, take Tates Creek Road/KY 169 west 12.5 miles to Valley View Ferry. To reach the put-in from the take-out, backtrack to Richmond, then join KY 52 East for 19 miles to the bridge over the Kentucky River, turning right to the river access before crossing the Kentucky River.

✧ **GAUGE** The USGS gauge is Kentucky River at Lock 14/Heidelberg. The minimum reading should be 600 cfs.

GPS COORDINATES

ACCESS	LATITUDE	LONGITUDE
F	N37° 41.836'	W83° 58.536'
G	N37° 47.052'	W84° 6.153'
H	N37° 51.200'	W84° 4.820'
I	N37° 51.723'	W84° 9.753'
J	N37° 53.277'	W84° 14.296'
K	N37° 53.277'	W84° 14.296'
L	N37° 52.984'	W84° 20.470'
M	N37° 51.460'	W84° 25.519'
N	N37° 50.807'	W84° 26.112'

Kentucky River Below the Forks: Irvine to Valley View Ferry

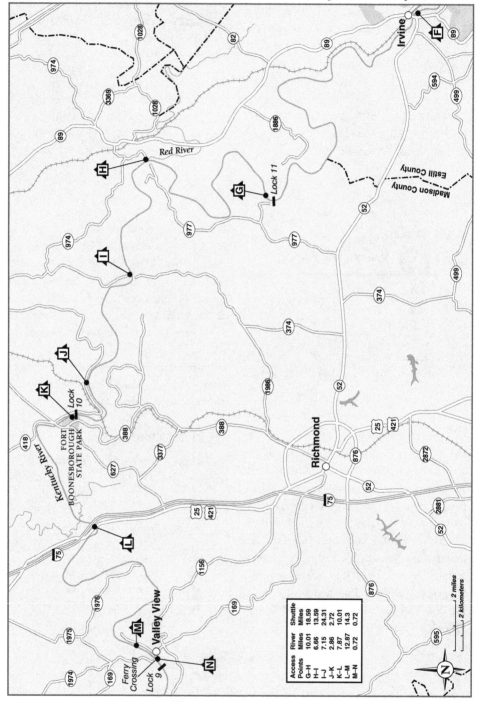

Access Points	River Miles	Shuttle Miles
G–H	10.01	18.59
H–I	6.66	13.59
I–J	7.15	24.31
J–K	2.86	2.72
K–L	7.87	10.01
L–M	12.87	14.3
M–N	0.72	0.72

D Lock 6 to Kentucky River View Park

Class I
Gauge Web
Level Min. 800– Max. flood (cfs)
Gradient 1'
Scenery B

see map on p. 70

16D DESCRIPTION The river averages 110–135 feet wide. This section has one lock to portage, Lock 5, above Clifton. It is 17 miles from Lock 6 to Lock 5, and 19 more miles to Frankfort.

SHUTTLE To reach the lowermost access in Frankfort, take US 421 North, Wilkinson Boulevard, from US 127 to Kentucky River View Park, which has a small boat launch. To reach the put-in from the take-out, return to US 127 and head south 23 miles. Turn left onto KY 1987 and follow it 2.2 miles to the put-in.

GAUGE The USGS gauge is Kentucky River at Lock 10/Winchester. The minimum reading should be 800 cfs.

GPS Coordinates

ACCESS	LATITUDE	LONGITUDE
V	N37° 55.556'	W84° 49.255'
W	N37° 58.398'	W84° 49.159'
X	N38° 2.044'	W84° 50.127'
Y	N38° 3.183'	W84° 49.778'
Z	N38° 4.640'	W84° 49.985'
AA	N38° 12.269'	W84° 52.729'

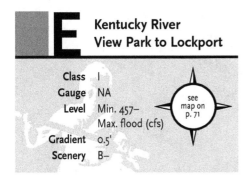

E Kentucky River View Park to Lockport

Class I
Gauge NA
Level Min. 457– Max. flood (cfs)
Gradient 0.5'
Scenery B–

see map on p. 71

16E DESCRIPTION Below Frankfort, the Kentucky River continues through farm valleys bordered by steep ridges. The level of difficulty remains Class I. Access is generally good. An outfitter is located at the confluence with Elkhorn Creek (EE). Lock 4 is just below the put-in, and Lock 3 is near Monterey (FF). The best access is on the east side of the river. These locks are in operation during the warm months. Double check the Kentucky River Authority's website for the latest on the locks at finance.ky.gov /offices/kra before paddling through this area.

SHUTTLE From Frankfort, take US 127 North to KY 355. Turn left and take KY 355 North to Gratz and KY 22. Turn left and take KY 22 West to KY 389 South. Turn left on KY 389 South and follow it to Lock 2. A boat ramp is just above the lock. To reach the uppermost access in Frankfort, take US 421 North, Wilkinson Boulevard, from US 127 to Kentucky River View Park, which has a small boat launch.

GAUGE The locks make the river runnable year-round. The normal pool stage for below Lock 4 is 457.1 feet.

GPS Coordinates

ACCESS	LATITUDE	LONGITUDE
BB	N38° 11.840'	W84° 52.747'
CC	N38° 12.269'	W84° 52.729'
DD	N38° 13.139'	W84° 52.633'
EE	N38° 13.139'	W84° 52.633'
FF	N38° 25.028'	W84° 52.724'
GG	N38° 26.346'	W84° 57.797'

(Continued on page 72)

Kentucky River Below the Forks: Lock 6 to Kentucky River View Park

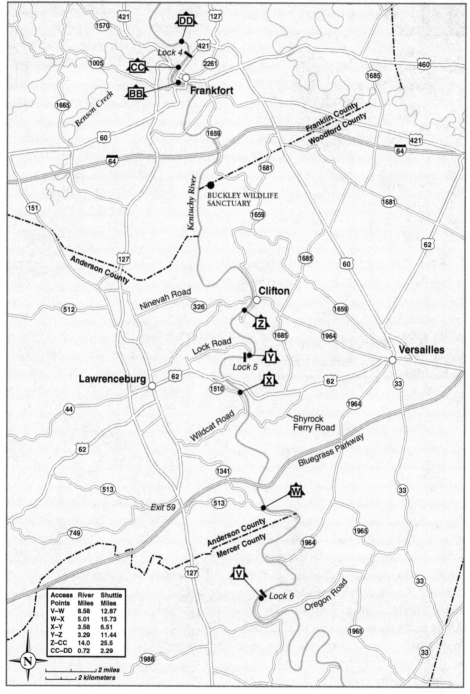

Access Points	River Miles	Shuttle Miles
V–W	8.58	12.87
W–X	5.01	15.73
X–Y	3.58	6.51
Y–Z	3.29	11.44
Z–CC	14.0	25.5
CC–DD	0.72	2.29

Kentucky River Below the Forks: Kentucky River View Park to Lockport

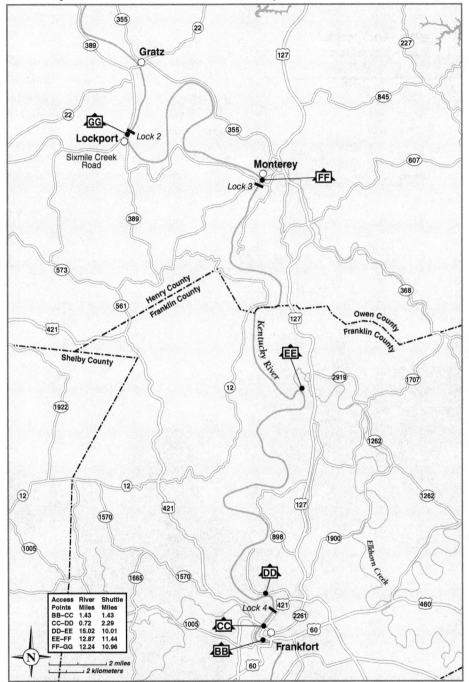

Access Points	River Miles	Shuttle Miles
BB–CC	1.43	1.43
CC–DD	0.72	2.29
DD–EE	15.02	10.01
EE–FF	12.87	11.44
FF–GG	12.24	10.96

(Continued from page 69)

F Lockport to Carrollton Boat Dock

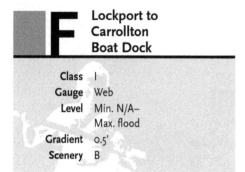

Class	I
Gauge	Web
Level	Min. N/A– Max. flood
Gradient	0.5'
Scenery	B

16F **DESCRIPTION** The Kentucky River is at its widest and largest here, ranging from 140 to 200 feet. Lock 1 is just above Carrollton. The take-out is on the Ohio River, upstream of the mouth of the Kentucky River, in historic Carrollton.

GAUGE The USGS gauge is Kentucky River at Lock 2/Lockport. However, the locks keep the river runnable all year.

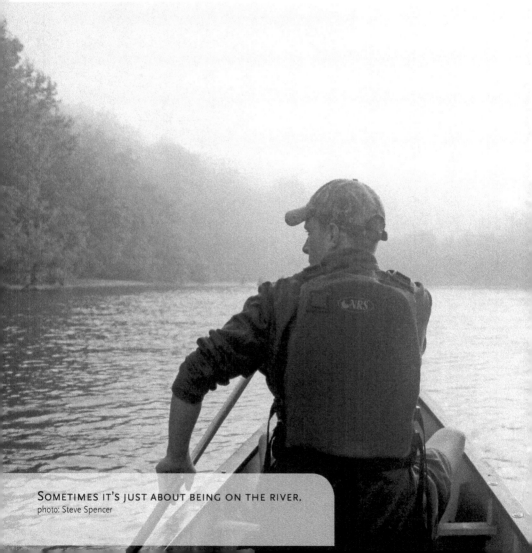

SOMETIMES IT'S JUST ABOUT BEING ON THE RIVER.
photo: Steve Spencer

Kentucky River Below the Forks: Lockport to Carrollton Boat Dock

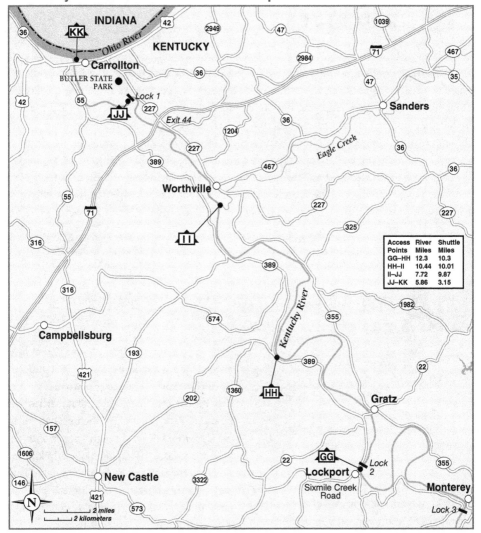

Access Points	River Miles	Shuttle Miles
GG–HH	12.3	10.3
HH–II	10.44	10.01
II–JJ	7.72	9.87
JJ–KK	5.86	3.15

GPS Coordinates

ACCESS	LATITUDE	LONGITUDE	ACCESS	LATITUDE	LONGITUDE
GG	N38° 26.346'	W84° 57.797'	JJ	N38° 39.488'	W85° 8.725'
HH	N38° 30.299'	W85° 1.731'	KK	N38° 41.003'	W85° 11.176'
II	N38° 35.779'	W85° 4.397'			

17 RED RIVER

◇ **OVERVIEW** Originating in Wolfe County, the Red River, Kentucky's only federally designated Wild and Scenic River, flows northwest through Powell County and along the Estill–Clark County line before emptying into the Kentucky River south of Winchester. During the early 1970s, national attention was focused on the river and on the beautiful Red River Gorge through which it flows, when Kentuckians and conservationists from throughout the country successfully fought the U.S. Army Corps of Engineers over the building of a dam. Hanging in the balance as the battle raged was the heart of the Red River and some of the most spectacular canoeing waters anywhere in the eastern United States. For paddling purposes, the Red River is popularly divided into three sections: the Upper, the Middle, and the Lower Red River.

◇ **MAPS** LEE CITY, CANNEL CITY, HAZEL GREEN, POMEROYTON, SLADE, STANTON, CLAY CITY, PALMER (USGS); DANIEL BOONE NATIONAL FOREST MAP, NORTH SECTION

A Upper Red River

Class	II (III)
Gauge	Web
Level	Min. 200–Max. 350/ 1,000 open/decked (cfs)
Gradient	13.29'
Scenery	A+

17A **DESCRIPTION** The Upper Red River is a Class II–III whitewater stream of unparalleled beauty winding among boulders and beneath cavernous overhangs. Only 20 feet wide at the put-in near the Big Branch access, the Upper Red remains intimate throughout, with hardwoods shading the water and mountain laurel growing thick above the rock ledges. The first 3 miles are scenic Class I water with a good current and a few small riffles and ledges. Below the mouth of Stillwater Creek, the gradient increases with a technical Class II rapid.

From here downstream the Red winds below imposing bluffs, assuming a pattern of alternating pools and small rapids (Class I+),

with the only interruption coming in the form of a river-wide ledge ranging from 1.5 to 3 feet in height and often referred to as the Falls. This ledge is sometimes difficult to get over at low to moderate water levels and is best run far left or far right. Continuing downstream, the river remains well behaved until it reaches the mouth of Peck Branch. For the next half mile, the Upper Red twists through a series of three borderline Class III rapids, popularly known as the Narrows of the Red. The first rapid is a long series of ledges with a healthy sampling of rocks to dodge, ending with a 2.5-foot plunge into a beautiful pool. Enter at the top left center, skirt the obstructing rocks as the water level allows, and pull into the eddy behind the last midstream rock before the vertical drop. Run the vertical drop by hugging the large boulder on the far left. The second rapid, 30 yards downstream, is known as Dog Drowning Hole and should probably be scouted (on the right). It consists of a turning chute accompanied by a great deal of turbulence. At low water it is very technical, and at higher water very squirrelly with irregular waves and currents. The total drop along the length of this

Red River: Upper Red River

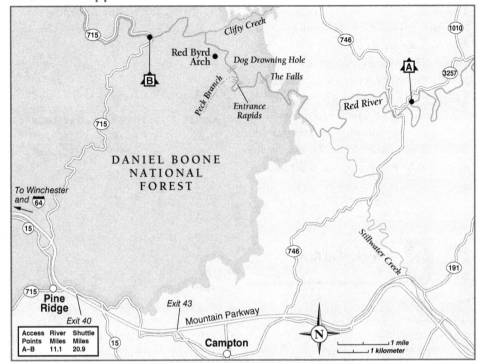

rapid is approximately 5 feet. At the third rapid of the Narrows, the river appears to come to a dead end. The current is deflected along the upstream face of a large boulder to the left bank, where it cuts right, down a fast sluice with an inclined 3-foot drop, finally washing up on an undercut rock 30 feet downstream. Run the sluice right center and grab an eddy on the right before the undercut rock grabs you. From here downstream to the take-out at the KY 715 bridge, the run is an easy Class II with delightful scenery and lots of hikers and backpackers at whom to wave.

The Upper Red is runnable from late December to late May in years of average rainfall. At very low water, the run can turn into a hike; however, the now-established USGS gauge at Hazel Green should eliminate most treks. At very high water, the Red is extremely dangerous, practically running in the trees, and only very experienced boating teams should enter the waters. Rapids on the Red are not especially difficult, but on the other hand, they allow little margin for error. Dangers other than those already described include frequent deadfalls, several undercut rocks, and the potential of the river to rise rapidly following a rain. The best time to run the Upper Red is in the morning because of the afternoon sun that shines directly into your eyes after about 2 p.m. An emergency walk-out exit can be found on river right shortly after the Falls of the Red. Look for the steel cables from an old swinging bridge over the river. Here, a rough path leads north out of the gorge onto farmland.

◇ **SHUTTLE** From Exit 40 on Mountain Parkway, take KY 15 North toward Slade to KY 715. Turn right and head north on KY 715 down to the Copperas Creek River Access on the Red. A national forest parking fee is required here. To reach the put-in from Exit 43 on Mountain Parkway, take KY 15 South to KY 191 East. Keep on KY 191 through Campton to reach KY 746. Turn right and follow KY 746 North past the bridge over the Red to KY 3357, Sandfield Road. Turn right on Sandfield Road and look for a signed right turn onto a gravel road and the Big Branch River Access. Do not use the KY 746 bridge for an access, as it is posted.

✧ **GAUGE** The USGS gauge is Red River near Hazel Green. The minimum reading should be 200 cfs.

GPS Coordinates

ACCESS	LATITUDE	LONGITUDE
A	N37° 48.147'	W83° 29.040'
B	N37° 49.232'	W83° 34.576'

B Middle Red River

Class	I+
Gauge	Web
Level	Min. 180–Max. flood (cfs)
Gradient	2.5'
Scenery	A

17B **DESCRIPTION** The middle section of the Red River begins at KY 715 bridge and twists through the center of the Red River Gorge; past Sky Bridge Arch, Tower Rock, and Chimney Top Rock; and works its way between boulders in the stream, eventually ending in the shadow of Raven Rock at the KY 77 bridge. Its level of difficulty is Class I throughout, but numerous sharp turns, sandbars, riffles, and small ledges make the paddling interesting. The scenery is spectacular without exception, with enormous hardwoods shading the stream and wildflowers in abundance. The middle section of the Red is runnable from late fall to early summer most years. Access is excellent. Navigational hazards consist of deadfalls, occasional logjams, and periodic overcrowding.

✧ **SHUTTLE** To reach the take-out from Exit 33 on the Bert T. Combs Mountain Parkway near Stanton, take KY 11 North 0.2 mile. Turn right onto KY 77 North and follow it 5.9 miles to the take-out at the bridge over the Red River. To reach the put-in from the take-out, keep east on KY 77 North, then join KY 715 East for 7 miles to the access just before the bridge crossing the Red River.

✧ **GAUGE** The USGS gauge is Red River at Clay City. The minimum reading should be 180 cfs.

GPS Coordinates

ACCESS	LATITUDE	LONGITUDE
B	N37° 49.232'	W83° 34.576'
C	N37° 50.004'	W83° 39.595'

Red River: Middle Red River

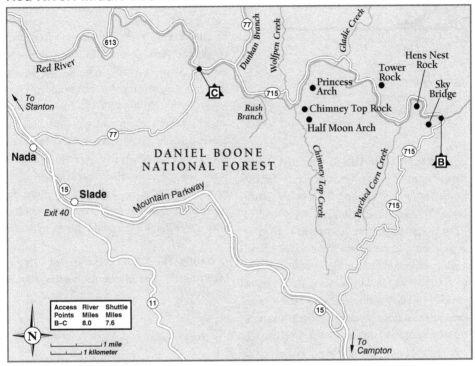

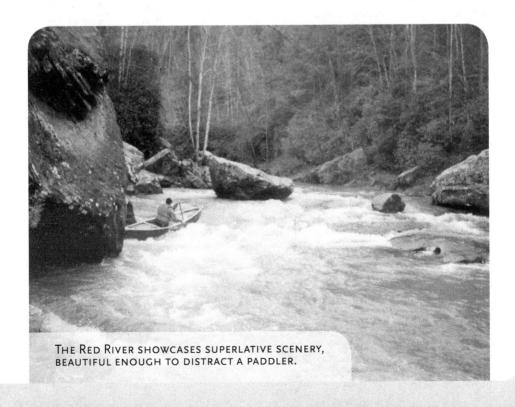

THE RED RIVER SHOWCASES SUPERLATIVE SCENERY, BEAUTIFUL ENOUGH TO DISTRACT A PADDLER.

C Lower Red River

Class	I
Gauge	Web
Level	Min. 180–Max. flood (cfs)
Gradient	2.5'
Scenery	B

17C **DESCRIPTION** The Lower Red River, downstream of KY 77, remains scenic for the first several miles, winding along below Courthouse Rock and finally running out of the Red River Gorge. From here downstream, the river is pleasant and meanders through hilly farm country and woodlands, but it does not compare to the upper and middle sections. Additionally, the lower section is almost always clogged with deadfalls that force portaging or swinging continually back and forth across the river to navigate around them. Flowing over a bed of gravel and mud between steep banks, the Lower Red is bordered by private property and is not suitable for camping. However, access points are numerous from bridges aplenty crossing the Red, availing day trips of varied lengths. Aside from deadfalls and logjams, there are no other navigational hazards. The Lower Red River averages 35–55 feet in width and is runnable from late fall to early summer.

◇ **SHUTTLE** To reach the take-out from Exit 16 on the Bert Combs Mountain Parkway, west of Stanton, briefly take KY 82 South, then turn right onto KY 1028 and go 4.9 miles. Turn right onto KY 3369 and follow it 2.6 miles. Turn left onto KY 974 West and follow it 0.1 mile. Turn left onto KY 89 South and travel 1.1 miles. Turn right onto Red River Road, go 0.8 mile, then stay straight as it becomes Ferry Road. Follow Ferry Road 1.1 miles to dead-end at the ramp at the confluence of the Red River and the Kentucky River.

◇ **GAUGE** The USGS gauge is Red River at Clay City, KY. The minimum reading should be 180 cfs.

GPS COORDINATES

ACCESS	LATITUDE	LONGITUDE
C	N37° 50.004'	W83° 39.595'
D	N37° 50.748'	W83° 46.128'
E	N37° 50.526'	W83° 48.525'
F	N37° 51.775'	W83° 51.312'
G	N37° 51.903'	W83° 56.003'
H	N37° 51.154'	W83° 57.007'
I	N37° 49.296'	W84° 4.175'
J	N37° 51.200'	W84° 4.820'

Red River: Lower Red River

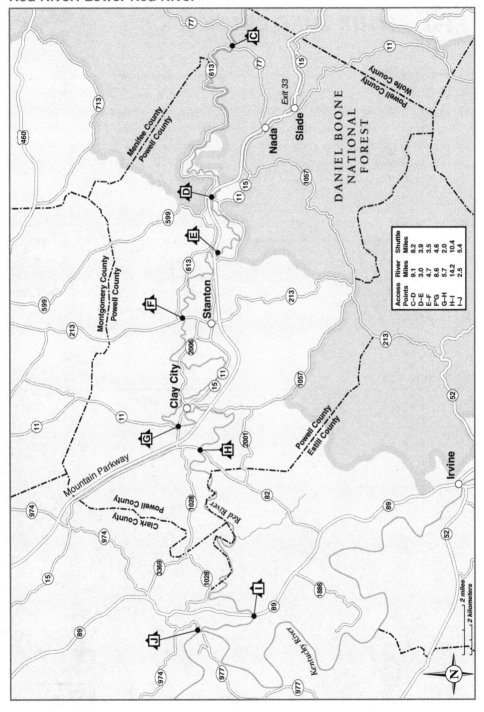

18 FOUR MILE CREEK

◇ **OVERVIEW** This is one of the first creeks to look for when the other whitewater creeks in the Clark/Madison County area are also running high. However, rains can be highly localized. The entire run is scoutable from the road and at moderate levels offers whitewater consisting of a very playful set of diagonal holes for the novice-intermediate boater. At higher levels this fast runoff stream contains numerous Class III hydraulics that will provide strong play boaters added fun and novices, increased trepidation.

◇ **MAPS** WINCHESTER (USGS)

Bybee Road to Kentucky River

Class	II–III (IV)
Gauge	Visual
Level	Min. 3"–Max. 2'
Gradient	40'
Scenery	A

◇ **DESCRIPTION** Much of the bank along the roadside of the creek has been concreted in, keeping the road from eroding away during high water but also making the creek seem like a drainage ditch. However, the creek itself is made up of numerous limestone ledges. The last half mile of the run is on the Kentucky River.

Four Mile Creek

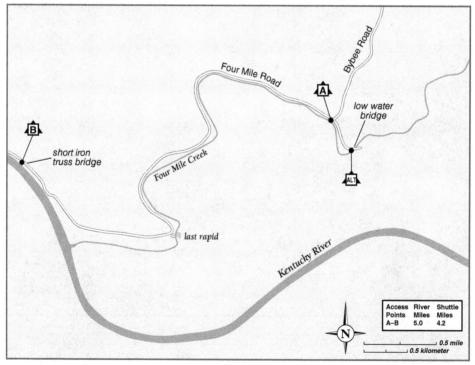

Four Mile Road

Bybee Road

A

low water
bridge

B

short iron
truss bridge

Four Mile Creek

ALT

last rapid

Kentucky River

Access Points	River Miles	Shuttle Miles
A–B	5.0	4.2

N

0.5 mile
0.5 kilometer

✧ **SHUTTLE** To reach Four Mile Creek from Winchester, take KY 1923 West to Bybee Road. Continue forward on Bybee Road until it comes to a T intersection at Four Mile Road and Four Mile Creek. Put in here, or turn left to signed Dead End Road that leads to a ford on Four Mile Creek and the property of boater-friendly landowner Alice Rankin. To reach the take-out, backtrack from signed Dead End Road and follow Four Mile Road until it curves around to Kentucky River. Good parking and decent landing on the Kentucky River are available past a small iron truss bridge that spans a feeder branch of Kentucky River.

✧ **GAUGE** What you see is what you get. If Howards Creek is running, Four Mile Creek is most likely running.

GPS COORDINATES

ACCESS	LATITUDE	LONGITUDE
A	N37° 53.364'	W84° 11.567'
B	N37° 53.146'	W84° 13.799'

19 LOWER HOWARDS CREEK

✧ **OVERVIEW** Lower Howards Creek is one of central Kentucky's most beautiful, interesting, and historic whitewater streams. Running through a narrow, remote, and lush gorge, the stream features remains of eighteenth-century architecture, including stone mill races, pioneer houses, and mills. Furthermore, this stream boasts almost continuous Class II–III rapids and numerous play places from the put-in to the take-out.

✧ **MAPS** FORD, WINCHESTER (USGS)

Old Stone Church Road to Kentucky River

Class	II–III (IV)
Gauge	Visual
Level	Min. 3"–Max. 2'
Gradient	40'
Scenery	A

see map on p. 82

✧ **DESCRIPTION** Even with its copious whitewater attributes, Lower Howards Creek is not a run for paddlers with weak rolls, who lack of precision boat control, or who are inattentive to downstream hazards. Even at moderate flows of 1 foot over the road, Howards could be upgraded to a solid Class IV stream with many blind turns; small, infrequent eddies; as well as numerous and ever-changing deadfalls, strainers, fences, and cables that require multiple portages.

✧ **SHUTTLE** To reach the take-out from Exit 96 on I-64, north of Winchester, take US 627 South to KY 418. Turn left and take KY 418 West under KY 627 Bridge to Halls Restaurant. Park here. To reach the put-in, backtrack to KY 627 and head north back to Old Stone Church Road. Turn left on Old Stone Church Road and follow it to a low-water bridge over Howards Creek. Do not block roads or cross the bridge at the parking area.

Lower Howards Creek

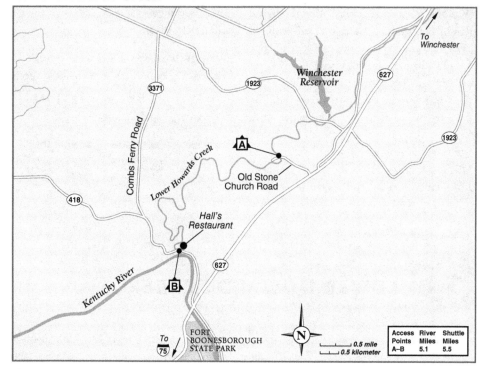

⟨⟩ GAUGE The gauge is where Old Stone Church Road crosses Lower Howards Creek. Minimum level is 3 inches of water over the road; maximum is 2 feet of water over the road.

GPS COORDINATES

ACCESS	LATITUDE	LONGITUDE
A	N37° 56.365'	W84° 14.647'
B	N37° 55.111'	W84° 16.389'

20 BOONE CREEK

⟨⟩ OVERVIEW Boone Creek is a small, intense stream flowing over a rock bed along the eastern border of Fayette County. Runnable only 10 or 12 days a year, it just may be the most singularly beautiful run in the entire state. The upper section (above the Iroquois Hunt Club) snakes over ledges between 20-foot-high rock walls. Passing the hunt club, Boone Creek's gradient increases as it descends into a narrow, vertical-walled rock gorge that funnels the stream at furious speed toward its mouth at the Kentucky River. Frequently, the constricting gorge walls recede, permitting trees to grow along the water's edge. At higher water levels, these trees create the only eddies on the run. Feeder streams join Boone Creek at several points below the hunt club. Two of these enter the creek after dropping over large waterfalls that are easily visible from Boone Creek. During the spring, wildflowers, particularly bluebells, further enhance the beauty of the stream.

◇ **MAPS** CLINTONVILLE, FORD (USGS)

KY 418 to Kentucky River

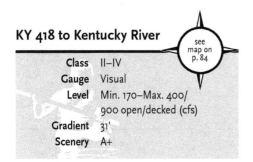

see map on p. 84

Class	II–IV
Gauge	Visual
Level	Min. 170–Max. 400/ 900 open/decked (cfs)
Gradient	31'
Scenery	A+

◇ **DESCRIPTION** Although Boone Creek may be beautiful, it is also dangerous. At higher water, it is a continuous Class III run (which some have classified as Class IV due to the scarcity of eddies). Its gradient averages 31 fpm but ranges as high as 44 fpm in certain sections. The gradient is evenly distributed, and no single drops exceeding 3 feet are encountered. Strainers in the form of deadfalls and logjams present the greatest danger. Creekwide farm fences may also occasionally appear in times of extended low water and then disappear completely or only partially be washed away in wet years. Fences are hazardous on any creek but particularly so on the Boone in light of the scarcity of eddies and the fast, pushy current at higher levels that allows very little time for the paddler to react. Action is continuous and consists primarily of standing waves, holes, and small drops, plus quick, twisting, and sometimes blind turns.

Boone Creek at high water is recommended only for experienced groups of two or more intermediate and advanced boaters with dependable rolls because rescue of swimming paddlers and their boats can be difficult among the vertical tree strainers. At moderate levels, Boone Creek is a good Class II to low Class III run. Parking at the KY 418 bridge put-in is limited to a small gravel road on river left downstream. Permission is generally given to park on the side of that road if you do not block it. Access at Grimes Mill Road Bridge near the Hunt Club (B) is not a good option; the area is signed as a no parking zone, and the Hunt Club and homeowners are hostile to anyone parking there. Parking is abundant at the take-out on KY 2328 (C). Dangers other than those mentioned include several undercut ledges. The last portion of the paddle is on the flatwater of the Kentucky River, which may back up a considerable distance into Boone Creek during times of high water.

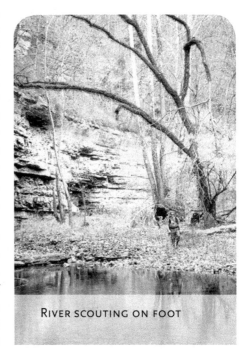

RIVER SCOUTING ON FOOT

✧ **SHUTTLE** To reach the take-out from Exit 99 on I-75, south of Richmond, take KY 2328/ Old Richmond Road 1.2 miles to the access on the Kentucky River. To reach the put-in from the take-out, backtrack on KY 2328, then join US 25 North and go 1.2 miles. Turn right onto McCalls Mill Road and follow it 2.4 miles. Turn right onto KY 418 and follow it 0.5 mile to the bridge and dirt road access.

✧ **GAUGE** Boone Creek is runnable only after heavy rains, more often in winter and spring.

GPS COORDINATES

ACCESS	LATITUDE	LONGITUDE
A	N37° 55.893'	W84° 20.381'
B	N37° 55.056'	W84° 20.480'
C	N37° 53.205'	W84° 20.340'

Boone Creek

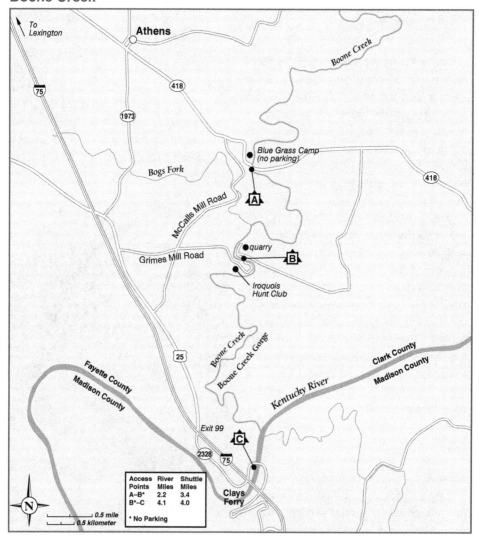

Access Points	River Miles	Shuttle Miles
A–B*	2.2	3.4
B*–C	4.1	4.0

* No Parking

0.5 mile
0.5 kilometer

21 HICKMAN CREEK

⟡ **OVERVIEW** East and West Fork Hickman flow forth from Lexington's two reservoirs and collect water as they run out of Lexington to Jessamine County. The creek offers some good central Kentucky scenery with woodland and farmland views, similar to those found on Elkhorn Creek (while being a smaller stream). However, Hickman is not as clean as the Elkhorn, in fact it can be downright poor, and the nice view is occasionally disrupted by trash along the creek banks.

⟡ **MAPS** LITTLE HICKMAN (USGS)

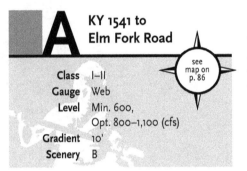

A KY 1541 to Elm Fork Road

see map on p. 86

Class	I–II
Gauge	Web
Level	Min. 600, Opt. 800–1,100 (cfs)
Gradient	10'
Scenery	B

21A DESCRIPTION This section is less exciting than most central Kentucky whitewater streams. It can be better described as a float. However, paddlers need to note a good wave just upstream of the Elm Fork Road Bridge. Check these surfing waves around 7–9 hours after the gauge reads 700–1,100 cfs. The best surfing water level is hard to catch: it becomes difficult to reach the wave when the water is really high, but when the water is low, it becomes less inviting.

⟡ **SHUTTLE** From Nicholasville, take KY 39 South for 3.7 miles, then turn left onto Elm Fork Road and follow it 2 miles to the take-out. To reach the put-in from the take-out, backtrack on Elm Fork Road 1.6 miles, then turn right onto West Lane and follow it 2 miles. Turn right onto KY 1541 and follow it 0.6 mile to the creek access.

⟡ **GAUGE** The virtual gauge used, on the American Whitewater website (americanwhitewater.org), is a combination of East and West Hickman Creeks and offers a quick resource to check the future creek level. However, to attain the most reliable prediction, consult and add the individual USGS gauges for East Hickman at Delong and West Hickman at Ashgrove Pike, using the fixed-width table output format for gauge reading and time. Both gauges are found above the commonly paddled sections and therefore are indicators of future flows. It usually takes 7–9 hours for the "virtual flow" to reach the take-out bridge on Elm Fork, although this will be affected by several factors beyond the scope of this description. The bare minimum reading is around 500 cfs for a float and 700 cfs for a park and surf. The maximum is around 1,500 cfs. Above 1,200 cfs, many of the best features begin to wash out and the creek takes on a flooded appearance.

GPS COORDINATES

ACCESS	LATITUDE	LONGITUDE
A	N37° 50.788'	W84° 30.517'
B	N37° 48.979'	W84° 32.255'

Hickman Creek: KY 1541 to Elm Fork Road

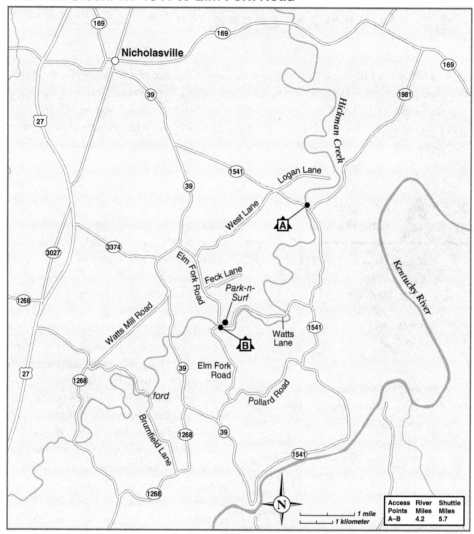

| | | 1 mile |
| | | 1 kilometer |

Access Points	River Miles	Shuttle Miles
A–B	4.2	5.7

B
Elm Fork Road to KY 1268 Bridge

Class	I–II (III)
Gauge	Web
Level	Min. 600; Opt. 800–1,100 (cfs)
Gradient	21'
Scenery	B

21B **DESCRIPTION** If you are in it purely for the whitewater, consider putting in at the ford on Brumfield Lane. Several rapids are just below this access, which is also a park-and-surf area. Your trip can be extended by putting in farther upstream at either Elm Fork Road, at Black Bridge on KY 39, or even at KY 1541. These longer trips will appeal to tandem canoeists, especially at lower water levels.

Hickman Creek: Elm Fork Road to KY 1268 Bridge

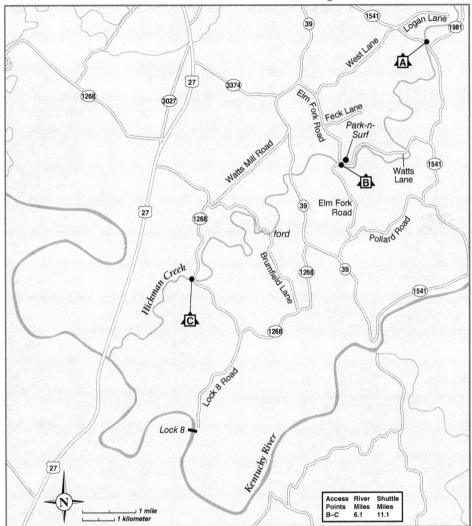

Access Points	River Miles	Shuttle Miles
B–C	6.1	11.1

⬦ SHUTTLE To reach the take-out from Nicholasville, take US 27 south to KY 1268 (it will be the second 1268 as you head south from Nicholasville). Turn left and take KY 1268 to the bridge over Hickman Creek. Parking is on the left, just before reaching the bridge. To reach the put-in, backtrack to Brumfield Lane, which may or may not be signed. It will be a very acute right-hand turn onto a paved road that looks like a driveway. Follow Brumfield Lane, passing Watts Mill Road, which veers left. (Watts Mill Road can be used to access upstream put-ins, as it cuts across KY 39 near additional stream crossings.) Keep on Brumfield Lane, and follow it to a wide, flat, low-water bridge over Hickman Creek. If the water is near the upper flow limits or rapidly rising, you must park on the hill before reaching the bottomland that surrounds the creek and road ford, which will be impassable when paddling is a possibility. Four-wheel drive, decent ground clearance, and pre–high water scouting are recommended.

◇ **GAUGE** The virtual gauge used, on the American Whitewater Association website (americanwhitewater.org), is a combination of East and West Hickman Creeks. Both gauges are found above the commonly paddled sections and therefore are indicators of future flows. It usually takes 8–10 hours for the "virtual flow" to reach the take-out bridge on KY 1268.

GPS Coordinates

ACCESS	LATITUDE	LONGITUDE
B	N37° 48.979'	W84° 32.255'
C	N37° 47.226'	W84° 35.128'

22 JESSAMINE CREEK

◇ **OVERVIEW** This stream offers a scenic paddle in close proximity to Nicholasville and south Lexington. It presents continuous twists and turns that are shrouded in overhanging trees and in the beginnings of a fairly deep gorge. There are also several interesting sites not found on other central Kentucky streams, including a postcard-scenic stone bridge at the take-out.

◇ **MAPS** WILMORE (USGS)

Frankfort Ford Road to KY 1268

Class	II (III)
Gauge	Visual
Level	N/A
Gradient	33'
Scenery	A–

◇ **DESCRIPTION** At low water, Jessamine can be scrapy, as many of the rapids are rock shoals rather than the typical central Kentucky limestone shelves. At high water, it offers decent excitement (II–II+ and maybe III when huge) and a few nice surfing waves that develop at differing water levels. There is a right turn rapid approximately a half mile into the trip, characterized by a rock outcropping that is fairly tight and could have a tendency to trap strainers. A couple other areas downstream are also narrow and could offer strainer traps and safety hazards. Additionally, there is a low-water road that crosses approximately halfway down from the put-in, and in the past there has been a chain stretched across the creek to keep drivers from venturing upstream at low water.

One rapid of note is very close to the take-out and is signaled by a right-hand rock wall and what appears to be a broken shelf or possibly an old dam or ford. With big water, this sloping area can create a couple of diagonal waves that make a paddler forget he or she is only in central Kentucky and offer quite a thrill. Also, there is a low-head dam (maybe 4–6 feet) just below the stone bridge at the take-out that is a safety hazard and bears mentioning. Although it has been run at medium flow, it could be very dangerous and offer a good chance of drowning, as low heads do. It is of note that the gorge downstream of this

Jessamine Creek

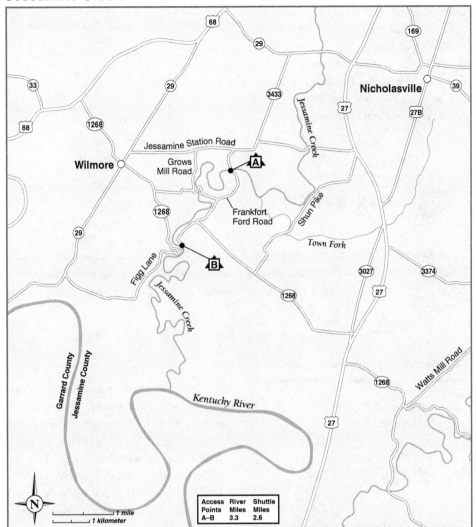

bridge is quite deep, with portions owned and reserved as conservation land. It is very scenic and offers significant eye and paddling appeal. However, access is limited, and it is therefore infrequently paddled.

◇ SHUTTLE To reach the take-out from Nicholasville, take US 27 South to KY 1268. Turn right on KY 1268 North and follow it to stop sign. Turn left at stop sign, staying with KY 1268, to reach a one-lane bridge over Jessamine Creek. Parking is very limited here. There is room for one car near the bridge and more room if you turn left onto Figg Lane, or continue on KY 1268, beyond the bridge. To reach the put-in, backtrack on KY 1268 to the stop sign. Continue forward past the stop sign, now on Frankfort Ford Road. Keep forward on Frankfort Ford Road to the bridge over Jessamine Creek.

⟡ **GAUGE** What you see is what you get. This creek runs only after heavy rains, particularly from late fall though spring leaf out. Jessamine Creek drains Nicholasville and surrounding developments, and takes a few hours to get from rainfall to put-in. That being said, several "viaducts" can be checked in downtown Nicholasville for a predictor of future flow.

GPS Coordinates

ACCESS	LATITUDE	LONGITUDE
A	N37° 51.564'	W84° 37.855'
B	N37° 50.541'	W84° 38.706'

23 DIX RIVER

⟡ **OVERVIEW** The Dix River originates in Rockcastle County and flows northwest through Lincoln County before being impounded to form Herrington Lake along the Garrard–Boyle County line. From the Dix River Dam, the river flows a short 2 miles before emptying into the Kentucky River.

⟡ **MAPS** Lancaster, Stanford, Bryantsvillle, Wilmore (USGS)

Logantown to Herrington Lake

Class	I++
Gauge	Web
Level	Min. 200–
	Max. flood (cfs)
Gradient	2.4'
Scenery	C+

⟡ **DESCRIPTION** Flowing primarily through farmland and wooded hills, the Dix is a pleasant, intimate river shaded by hardwoods and occasionally graced with some small bluffs and exposed rock ledges. Running over a mud bottom in the upper stretches between often-steep mud banks, the streambed changes to a rock bottom with boulders along the bank as the Dix approaches the mouth of the Hanging Fork. Its level of difficulty is Class I, although several tight spots require good boat control. Riffles, small ledges, and shoals are not uncommon.

Dangers to navigation consist mainly of deadfalls and occasional logjams. The Dix is runnable from late fall to late spring downstream of the US 27 bridge at Logantown (B). Other access points are KY 1150 (C) and KY 52 (D). Canoe camping is possible if adjoining sections of the river and lake are combined. Campgrounds are all privately owned and charge for camping space.

⟡ **SHUTTLE** To reach the take-out from Lancaster, take US 27 North 7 miles, then turn left onto KY 34 West and follow it 0.9 mile. Make a quick right onto County Road 1329, followed by an immediate left onto Kings Mill Road to reach privately owned Kings Mill Marina. To reach the put-in from the take-out, backtrack through Lancaster, following US 27 south for a total of 10.5 miles. Turn left onto Gilberts Creek Cutoff and follow it 1.2 miles. Turn

Dix River

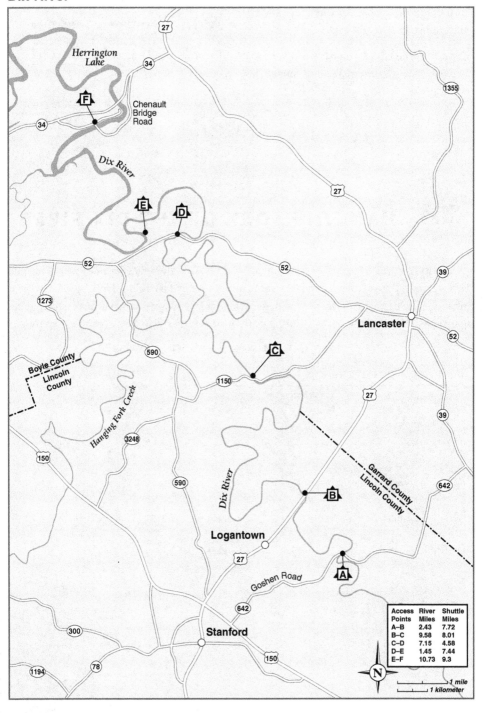

Access Points	River Miles	Shuttle Miles
A–B	2.43	7.72
B–C	9.58	8.01
C–D	7.15	4.58
D–E	1.45	7.44
E–F	10.73	9.3

right onto Patrick Road and travel 1.4 miles. Turn right onto Goshen Road and follow it 0.7 mile to the Dix River bridge.

✧ **GAUGE** The USGS gauge is Dix River near Danville, KY. Minimum reading should be 200 cfs.

GPS COORDINATES

ACCESS	LATITUDE	LONGITUDE
A	N37° 33.296'	W84° 36.196'
B	N37° 34.267'	W84° 36.987'
C	N37° 36.176'	W84° 38.088'
D	N37° 38.506'	W84° 39.680'
E	N37° 38.537'	W84° 40.366'
F	N37° 40.330'	W84° 41.448'

≈≈≈

24 HANGING FORK OF THE DIX RIVER

✧ **OVERVIEW** The Hanging Fork, a tributary of the Dix River flowing northeast along the Boyle–Lincoln County line, is runnable from late fall to early May below the KY 590 bridge. An interesting little stream (15–30 feet wide), the Hanging Fork twists through a small, shady gorge interrupted occasionally as grassy, grazing plains insinuate themselves between the steep ridges.

✧ **MAPS** STANFORD (USGS)

Hanging Fork of the Dix River

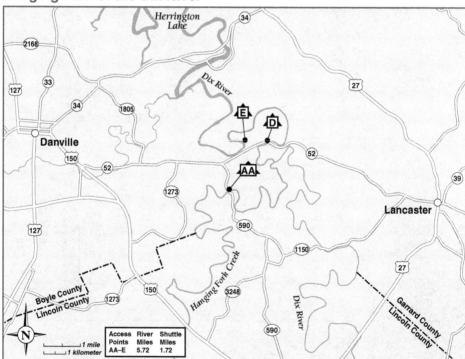

KY 590 to Dix River at KY 52

Class	I (II)
Gauge	Visual
Level	Min. 120–Max. 400 (cfs)
Gradient	14'
Scenery	B

◊ DESCRIPTION The paddling is rated a busy Class I and borderline Class II with almost continuous small shoals and rapids. There are numerous deadfalls and immense log-jams to avoid. Grass and brush is common around shoals. There is also a small dam near the confluence with the Dix that may be portaged or (at favorable water levels) run on the left, where the dam is partially collapsed. Scout first! Emerging on the Dix River, the take-out is three-quarters of a mile downstream below the confluence with the Dix at the KY 52 bridge.

◊ SHUTTLE To reach the take-out from Lancaster, take KY 52 West 5 miles to the dirt access on the left just before the bridge over the Dix River. To reach the put-in from the take-out, continue west on KY 52 for 1.4 miles. Turn left onto KY 590 and follow it 0.8 mile to the bridge over the Hanging Fork.

◊ GAUGE If the Dix is running high and the water looks floatable at the KY 590 bridge on the Hanging Fork, the trip should be a go.

GPS Coordinates

ACCESS	LATITUDE	LONGITUDE
AA	N37° 37.436'	W84° 40.799'
E	N37° 38.537'	W84° 40.366'

25 GILBERT CREEK

◊ OVERVIEW Gilbert Creek is an often-overlooked paddle stream, probably due to its small watershed. Draining the southeastern corner of Anderson County, south of Lawrenceburg, Gilbert Creek flows into the Kentucky River. Load your boat after a heavy rainfall of 2 inches or more during winter or early spring. Be forewarned: with a gradient of 75 feet per mile, this is for serious whitewater boaters only.

◊ MAPS McBrayer (USGS)

Gilbert Creek Road to Kentucky River

Class	II–III+	
Gauge	Visual	see map on p. 94
Level	N/A	
Gradient	75'	
Scenery	A	

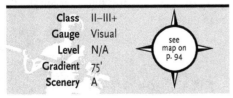

◊ DESCRIPTION This is not a creek for beginners. It starts fast and furious and never lets up. Limestone ledges are featured top to bottom. Because of its size and gradient, there are very few eddies. Take advantage of the shuttle to scout wherever you can. Much of the run can be scouted from the road. There are many trees to avoid, and it is likely you will encounter deadfalls. Boat scouting is possible, but everyone in the group will have to fend for themselves, because what eddies that do exist will fill up quickly with one or two boats.

Be ready for play spots at any time—there are numerous surf waves and ledge holes the length of the run. If in doubt at any of the larger ledges,

Gilbert Creek

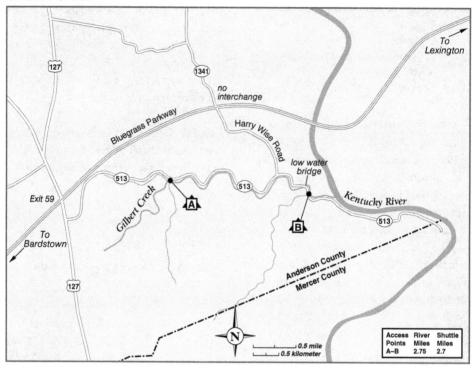

go left, where the current flushes out. The largest of the ledges is a 4-foot sloping ledge with a tongue on the left that is followed by a quick right turn. It can be seen from the road and is located just below a private bridge halfway along the run.

At about 2 miles, there will be a small creek entering from the left. Gilbert Creek will narrow and begin to accelerate down a 50-yard stretch with a constant gradient. Every ounce of the creek's energy will become focused as it enters a large pool. The result is a startlingly large haystack wave that you must crash through. Be alert for the take-out on the left—there is a very bad hydraulic below the low-water crossing.

◇ **SHUTTLE** From Exit 59 on the Blue Grass Parkway, take US 127 South just a short distance to KY 513. Turn left on KY 513 and follow it 2.7 miles, passing the private low-water

bridge put-in on the way (1156 address). Continue down KY 513 to the low-water bridge on KY 513 crossing Gilbert Creek. This is the take-out. From there, backtrack to the previously mentioned private low-water bridge and put-in.

◇ **GAUGE** The low-water bridge—visible from the Blue Grass Parkway and the first one you will see on your right heading along the creek—has pipes running under it. If the pipes are more than half full, then you should be in business.

GPS COORDINATES

ACCESS	LATITUDE	LONGITUDE
A	N37° 58.533'	W84° 51.173'
B	N37° 58.418'	W84° 49.496'

26 BENSON CREEK

✧ **OVERVIEW** Benson Creek flows northeast out of Anderson County, through Franklin County to the Kentucky River at Frankfort. Runnable above the confluence of the forks after heavy rains and below the confluence from late fall through the spring, Benson Creek offers a variety of surprises. The waterway is often floated by locals when the water is up, generally November to mid-May following heavy rains.

✧ **MAPS** Frankfort West (USGS)

KY 1005 to Benson Valley boat ramp

Class	II–III
Gauge	Visual
Level	Min. 3', above 5.5', experts only
Gradient	15.7'
Scenery	B+

✧ **DESCRIPTION** When it comes to whitewater play boating, some say, "go big or go home." Benson Creek can get big, during its 10–20 times per year of being runnable, and then only for 4–10 hours at a time. When runnable, the North Fork, below Sheep Pen Road, powers through fields and pastureland until suddenly it veers to the right and drops over

Benson Creek

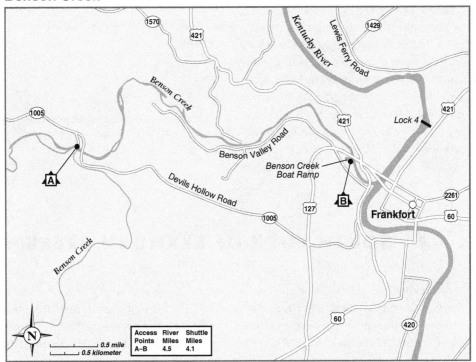

Access Points A–B   River Miles 4.5   Shuttle Miles 4.1

0.5 mile
0.5 kilometer

a 13-foot vertical falls. However, two of the biggest rapids on the creek are here. One rapid, Big Bitch, is a deep hole where paddlers can do almost any freestyle move capable in a hole, including aerial loops. Another wave above the falls, Big Slut, is the only aerial wave in Kentucky. This is more of a low to moderate water level feature that is prime around 3–4 feet. Big Bitch is prime above 4.5 feet.

The South Fork, averaging only 20 feet in width downstream of the Pea Ridge Road put-in, drops swiftly over Class I and II ledges. Too many hard-to-see cattle fences and a lack of eddies make this run too dangerous at any water level, no matter your level of expertise. The Falls of Benson should be run just left of center at moderate water levels.

Fortunately, Benson Creek below the confluence of the forks (just downstream of the large falls) is somewhat more predictable. Flowing between tall, beautiful, wooded bluffs (many with exposed rock), Benson Creek becomes a scenic and delightful Class II run with exceptional play boating river opportunities. Rapids consist primarily of river-wide ledges ranging from 1 to 3 feet in height that can be run just about anywhere. Holes occurring below the drops are generally friendly at most water levels. Several rapids disappear around curves and should be scouted for possible obstructions (deadfalls). Hazards include deadfalls, logjams, and a 5-foot low-head dam

at the distillery that should be portaged on the right. Some paddlers punch over the dam at one of two holes because there is no hydraulic. The final half mile or so of the run is on slack water before reaching the Benson Creek boat ramp.

⟡ **SHUTTLE** From downtown Frankfort, take US 127 South to KY 1211 South, then turn right on Benson Valley Road to reach the boat ramp on your right. To reach the put-in, return to US 127 and head south to turn right on Devils Hollow Connector and pick up KY 1005 West to reach the bridge over Benson Creek just below the falls. However, there are NO PARKING signs all around the bridge area, and tickets have been given for violation. The best option is to go upstream to access at KY 1665, where you can park across the railroad track on the side of the gravel road to the right.

⟡ **GAUGE** At the KY 1005 bridge, Devils Hollow Road, near the falls. Minimum runnable level is 3.0; above 5.5 is for expert boaters only.

GPS COORDINATES

ACCESS	LATITUDE	LONGITUDE
A	N38° 12.528'	W84° 56.275'
B	N38° 12.384'	W84° 53.172'

27   SOUTH FORK OF ELKHORN CREEK

⟡ **OVERVIEW** Similar to the North Fork of Elkhorn Creek, the South Fork of Elkhorn Creek is also very seasonal, being runnable mostly during the winter and spring. Tree lined and flowing through gently rolling terrain amidst fertile fields and picturesque Bluegrass horse farms, the South Fork can be paddled below (downstream of) Fishers Mill in Woodford County.

⟡ **MAPS** VERSAILLES, MIDWAY, FRANKFORT EAST, SWITZER (USGS)

South Fork of Elkhorn Creek

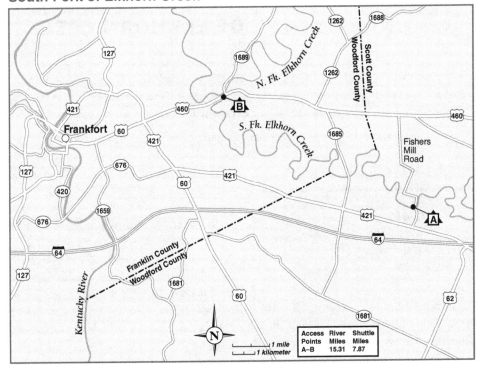

Access Points	River Miles	Shuttle Miles
A–B	15.31	7.87

Fishers Mill to Forks of Elkhorn

Class	I+
Gauge	Visual and phone
Level	Min. 125–Max. flood (cfs)
Gradient	1.4'
Scenery	B–

✧ **DESCRIPTION** An exceptionally winding stream with continually changing vistas, the South Fork of Elkhorn Creek sports a variety of small riffles and ledges to enliven the paddling. Access is limited, and the level of difficulty is Class I. Hazards to navigation include deadfalls and a large dam (portage right) near the confluence with the North Fork.

✧ **SHUTTLE** To reach the Forks of Elkhorn from Frankfort, take US 60 East to US 460. Keep east on US 460 to KY 460 to reach Scruggs Road and Elkhorn Campground and the take-out. To reach the put-in from the take-out, return to US 460 and follow it east 2.8 miles. Turn right onto KY 1685 and travel 2.6 miles. Turn left onto US 421 South and follow it 1.8 miles to Fishers Mill Road. Turn left onto Fishers Mill Road and reach the bridge over South Fork at 0.6 mile.

✧ **GAUGE** What you see is what you get. However, consider contacting Canoe Kentucky at the Forks of the Elkhorn for runnable level (502-227-4492, canoeky.com).

GPS COORDINATES

ACCESS	LATITUDE	LONGITUDE
A	N38° 10.422'	W84° 42.377'
B	N38° 12.899'	W84° 47.914'

28 NORTH FORK OF ELKHORN CREEK

✧ **OVERVIEW** The North Fork of Elkhorn Creek flows through Scott County and is runnable from late fall to late spring from Georgetown downstream. Several dams in the Georgetown vicinity create pools that permit the paddling of certain 2- to 4-mile stretches year-round.

✧ **MAPS** GEORGETOWN, MIDWAY, STAMPING GROUND, SWITZER (USGS)

KY 36 Bridge to Kentucky River

Class	I+
Gauge	Web
Level	Min. 180–Max. flood (cfs)
Gradient	4'
Scenery	B–

✧ **DESCRIPTION** By and large, the North Fork winds through rolling farmland, though suburban Georgetown has encroached onto the northern North Fork's shores. Trees line the mud and rock banks that vary markedly in height and steepness. The most popular run on the North Fork begins at the covered bridge near Switzer (F) and terminates at the confluence of the North and South Forks (G). In this stretch, the stream grows progressively rockier, and many small ledges and rapids appear (all Class I). Boat ramps near Georgetown make access good on the uppermost stream. Dangers to navigation include dams (as mentioned) that must be portaged and deadfalls. The dam just above KY 1688 has washed out and is now runnable. However, the access at KY 1688 (E) is tenuous due to adjacent landowners. The level of difficulty is

Class I throughout, the average width is 35–40 feet, and access is mostly good.

✧ **SHUTTLE** To reach the Forks of Elkhorn from Frankfort, take US 60 East to US 460. Keep east on US 460 to KY 460 to reach Scruggs Road and Elkhorn Campground and the take-out. To reach the uppermost put-in at Georgetown, continue on US 460 East to Georgetown and the bridge over North Fork. Look left, just after the bridge for Oser Landing Park.

✧ **GAUGE** The USGS gauge is Elkhorn Creek near Frankfort, KY. The minimum reading should be 180 cfs.

GPS COORDINATES

ACCESS	LATITUDE	LONGITUDE
A	N38° 12.797'	W84° 32.723'
B	N38° 13.248'	W84° 33.823'
C	N38° 12.967'	W84° 36.308'
D	N38° 13.959'	W84° 39.243'
E	N38° 14.743'	W84° 42.356'
F	N38° 15.239'	W84° 45.119'
G	N38° 12.899'	W84° 47.914'

North Fork of Elkhorn Creek

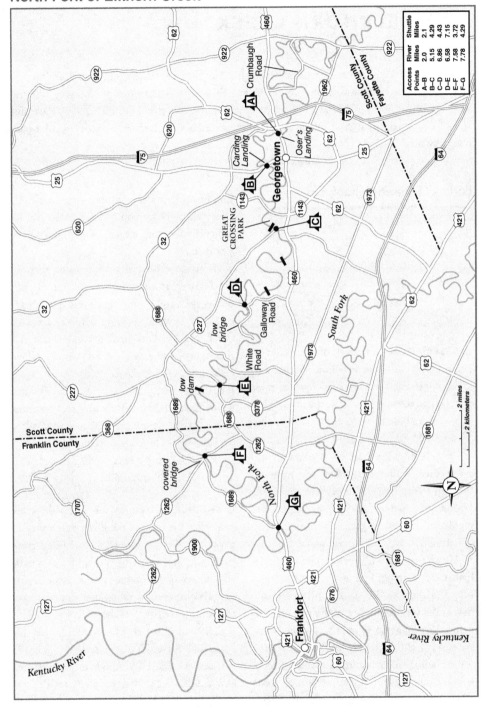

Access Points	River Miles	Shuttle Miles
A–B	2.0	2.1
B–C	5.15	4.29
C–D	6.86	4.43
D–E	6.58	7.15
E–F	7.58	3.72
F–G	7.78	4.29

29   ELKHORN CREEK

◇ **OVERVIEW** Elkhorn Creek, with its North and South Forks, flows northwest, draining portions of Jessamine, Fayette, Scott, Woodford, and Franklin Counties before emptying into the Kentucky River north of Frankfort. Because of its mild whitewater, beautiful scenery, plentiful access, and proximity to four major urban areas, the Elkhorn is Kentucky's most popular paddling stream.

◇ **MAPS** SWITZER, POLSGROVE (USGS)

Forks of Elkhorn to Kentucky River

Class	I+; whitewater section, II–III
Gauge	Web
Level	Min. 240–Max. 850/ flood open/decked (cfs)
Gradient	9.5'
Scenery	B

◇ **DESCRIPTION** Northeast of Frankfort at Forks of Elkhorn, the two forks of Elkhorn Creek come together. Here begins the most popular and scenic of the Elkhorn's many offerings: 6 miles of lively Class II and III whitewater. Runnable from late fall to early summer, this 6-mile stretch is a perfect training ground for novice whitewater paddlers. Running through a deep gorge with exposed rock walls (sometimes reaching 200 feet in height), the rapids, riffles, and ledges are almost continuous. In all, there are four legitimate Class III rapids on this run with perhaps six additional high Class I or borderline Class IIs. Several islands punctuate the stream. All except the first at the very beginning of the run are normally run along the right side. At low water, the run is technical and helpful in developing water-reading skills. At high water (3 feet), large standing waves predominate. Access is good. Dangers to navigation include a dam (mandatory portage, on left) adjacent to the

Jim Beam Distillery, low-hanging branches, and occasional logjams. This portage can be difficult when the stream is running above 3,000 cfs.

Downstream of the whitewater section, the Elkhorn is runnable year-round. It continues swift and beautiful, flowing over a rock bed as it moves toward its rendezvous with the Kentucky. This final section clears the rocky gorge and drops into an intimate valley. Ledges, riffles, and small rapids persist, as do some more, fairly large islands. The stream's width fluctuates widely in this section from a constricting 35 feet to a broad and shallow 90 feet. Access is good, and deadfalls and logjams are the only navigational dangers. The level of difficulty is Class I.

◇ **SHUTTLE** The put-in for the whitewater run below the forks of the Elkhorn is a private pay put-in (G). It is at the KY 460 bridge, river right, just upstream of the bridge. To park and put-in at the bridge, pay at the Elkhorn Creek Campground office just upstream on the South Fork of the Elkhorn.

Take-out for the whitewater run is on Peaks Mill Road, KY 1900, and (H). There is a take-out owned by American Whitewater (AW), donated by local paddlers, on the left just before Knight's Bridge over the Elkhorn. An additional landing has been established by

Elkhorn Creek

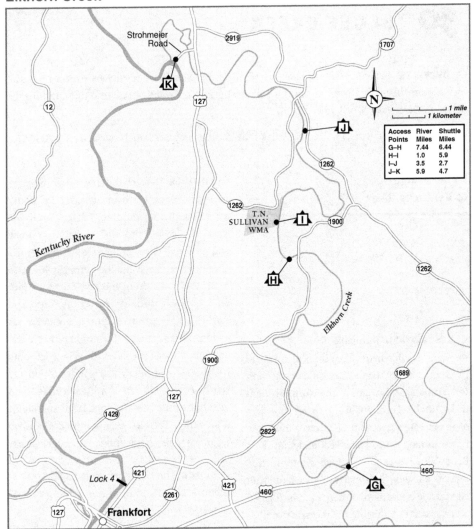

Access Points	River Miles	Shuttle Miles
G–H	7.44	6.44
H–I	1.0	5.9
I–J	3.5	2.7
J–K	5.9	4.7

Kentucky Fish and Wildlife a little downstream of the AW take-out, at T. N. Sullivan Wildlife Management Area, off Sullivan Lane, KY 1262 (I). Canoe Kentucky has a pay access on the east bank upstream of the Peaks Mill Bridge (J).

✧ **GAUGE** The USGS gauge is Elkhorn Creek near Frankfort, KY. The minimum reading should be 240 cfs.

GPS COORDINATES

ACCESS	LATITUDE	LONGITUDE
G	N38° 12.899'	W84° 47.914'
H	N38° 16.060'	W84° 49.000'
I	N38° 18.356'	W84° 48.882'
J	N38° 19.149'	W84° 49.582'
K	N38° 19.040'	W84° 51.250'

30   EAGLE CREEK

◇ **OVERVIEW** Eagle Creek originates in Scott County and flows northwest over a mud and rock bottom through Owen, Grant, Carroll, and Gallatin Counties before emptying into the Kentucky River near Worthville.

◇ **MAPS** LAWRENCEVILLE, ELLISTON, GLENCOE, SANDERS, VEVAY SOUTH, WORTHVILLE (USGS)

KY 36 Bridge to Kentucky River

Class	I+
Gauge	Web
Level	Min. 190–Max. flood
Gradient	4.7'
Scenery	C

◇ **DESCRIPTION** Runnable from November through May downstream of the KY 36 bridge in Grant County, Eagle Creek flows through the farmland and woods of the Northern Kentucky Knobs. Throughout the upper stretches of the stream (upstream of Sparta), the Eagle flows through a broad and frequently saturated floodplain. Banks are inclined gently in this section allowing seasonal rains to flatten all streamside vegetation. Brush islands formed on river curves following the recession of high water are common and provide navigational challenge to the paddler.

Below (downstream of) Sparta (F), the 45-foot stream runs more deeply as steeper banks channel the flow, and some very small ledges and rapids are encountered. The banks are tree lined all along the Eagle but very thinly so. The level of difficulty is Class I throughout, with deadfalls being the foremost danger to paddlers. Access is excellent between the KY 36 bridge and Worthville. The preferred access near Worthville is on the Kentucky River (I).

◇ **SHUTTLE** To reach the take-out from Exit 71 on I-71 north of Worthville, take KY 227 South 4.8 miles. Turn right onto KY 355 South and travel 0.7 mile. Turn right onto River Road and go 1 mile to reach the ramp at the confluence of Eagle Creek and the Kentucky River. To reach the put-in from the take-out, backtrack on River Road, turn right on KY 355 South, and stay with it for 4.7 miles. Turn left onto KY 325 and follow it 5.6 miles. Turn right onto KY 227 South and travel 2.3 miles, then veer left onto KY 36 East and follow it 2.9 miles to US 127 North. Follow US 127 North for 1 mile, then turn right onto Stewart Ridge Road and follow it 4.5 miles. Turn left onto KY 36 East and go 3.9 miles to reach the bridge over Eagle Creek.

◇ **GAUGE** The USGS gauge is Eagle Creek at Glencoe, KY. The minimum reading should be 190.

GPS COORDINATES

ACCESS	LATITUDE	LONGITUDE
A	N38° 38.650'	W84° 42.852'
B	N38° 40.565'	W84° 45.134'
C	N38° 41.129'	W84° 45.201'
D	N38° 42.904'	W84° 44.973'
E	N38° 42.348'	W84° 49.547'
F	N38° 40.616'	W84° 54.303'
G	N38° 39.028'	W84° 56.704'
H	N38° 36.177'	W85° 4.102'
I	N38° 35.775'	W85° 4.392'

Eagle Creek

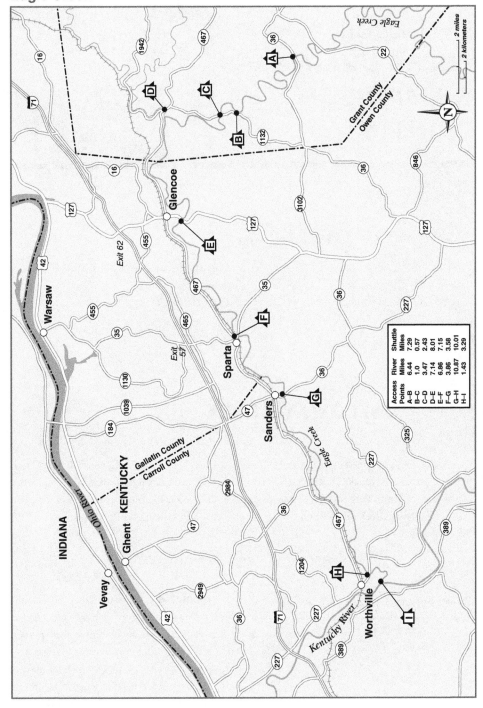

Access Points	River Miles	Shuttle Miles
A–B	6.44	7.29
B–C	1.0	0.57
C–D	3.47	2.43
D–E	7.14	8.01
E–F	6.86	7.15
F–G	3.86	3.58
G–H	10.87	10.01
H–I	1.43	3.29

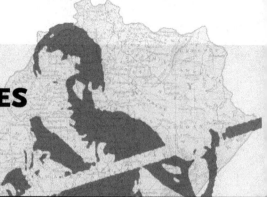

PART FOUR
CREEK DRAINAGES OF MADISON COUNTY

31 CALLOWAY CREEK

✧ **OVERVIEW** This creek is also referred to—erroneously—as Galloway Creek. Calloway Creek plunges into the Kentucky River near the I-75 bridge south of Lexington. Runnable below the confluence of Smith Fork, this creek was first descended by local Kentucky paddlers in the early 2000s. Calloway Creek ranks as one of the most scenic and intense whitewater streams in the Bluegrass State.

✧ **MAPS** Ford, Richmond North (USGS)

Smith Fork to Kentucky River

Class	II–IV
Gauge	Visual
Level	Min. N/A–Max. N/A
Gradient	80'
Scenery	A+

✧ **DESCRIPTION** Calloway Creek boasts numerous nonstop, steep, vertical, and chaotic Class IV slide-style rapids through a spectacular high-walled canyon. Be watchful for cross-creek cattle fences that an alert paddler may be able to pass under, depending on flow levels. Also, be apprised of creek-wide tree strainers.

Calloway Creek

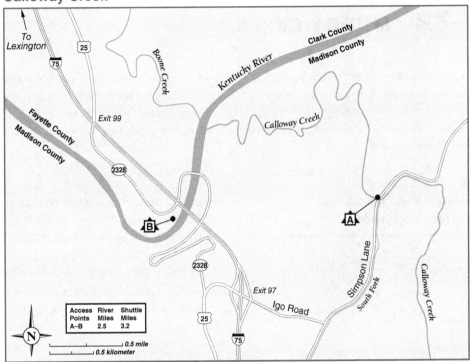

First-time paddlers of Calloway should possess good boat scouting skills or should follow a Calloway veteran because there are numerous horizon lines with poor bank scouting possibilities. Calloway Creek enters the Kentucky River directly across from Boone Creek. The last part of the paddle is on the Kentucky River.

⬦ **SHUTTLE** From Exit 99 on I-75 south of Lexington, take KY 2328 South to the bridge over the Kentucky River. To reach the put-in from the take-out, continue south on KY 2328 for 1.6 miles. Turn left onto US 25 North, then keep straight, crossing the interstate and joining Igo Road for 0.5 mile; then turn left onto Simpson Lane. Follow Simpson Lane 0.9 mile to reach the bridge of Smith Fork entering Calloway Creek and a put-in.

⬦ **GAUGE** There is no gauge for Calloway Creek, but this stream can be visually checked following a significant rain event that brings the rest of Madison County's whitewater streams into runnable levels.

GPS COORDINATES

ACCESS	LATITUDE	LONGITUDE
A	N37° 53.092'	W84° 19.028'
B	N37° 52.984'	W84° 20.460

32 MUDDY CREEK

◆ **OVERVIEW** Muddy Creek is considered by many to be the best whitewater play stream in central Kentucky. With a drainage area of 63 square miles, Muddy Creek usually has a lag time of 3 hours or more following a heavy rain and will typically remain running for 12–24 hours. If you are able to run Tates Creek or any of the branches of Otter Creek, then the Muddy is probably flowing as well.

◆ **MAPS** UNION CITY, MOBERLY (USGS)

Oakley Wells Road Bridge to near Doylesville

Class	II (III)
Gauge	Visual
Level	Min. N/A–Max. N/A
Gradient	20'
Scenery	B

◆ **DESCRIPTION** Although it lacks any single, large drop or difficult rapid, Muddy Creek provides more surfing/freestyle fun per mile than any other whitewater run in the Bluegrass. Several small waterfalls add to the scenic quality of this run, which consists of mostly Class II–III easy and wide-open rapids, with the very first rapid being the most difficult of the run. The Muddy contains hundreds of small ledges, forming essentially nonstop surfing waves and holes along its entire length. Many drops offer no-wait surfing for even for the largest of paddling groups. A river-wide hydraulic in the upper third of the run has several surfing boaters at once, confirming its name of Five Boat Hole. There is also a nice, single hydraulic park and surf in sight of the bridge where Cane Springs Road crosses the creek. At levels above "suck" (see gauge info), the Muddy tends to wash out, losing its great surfing. Hazards include the standard: strainers, brush piles, and floating debris.

◆ **SHUTTLE** To reach the put-in, take KY 52 East from Richmond to KY 977. Turn left and take KY 977 to Oakley Wells Road. The normal put-in can be reached by following Oakley Wells Road around the right-angle turn at the put-in. Do not go straight downstream on the dirt/gravel lane; that is a private drive. Park adjacent to the private drive on Oakley Wells Road. To reach the take-out, head west on Oakley Wells Road to Charlie Norris Road and turn right into beautiful downtown Union City. Turn right again at the small market onto KY 1986, the Union City Expressway, and follow it into Doylesville. Here, KY 1986 makes two 90-degree bends—first right, then left; keep forward on a dead-end road, as Weddles Mill Road turns right. Reach a bridge over Muddy Creek. Park in the gravel area on the left of the bridge before crossing the bridge. If you cross Muddy Creek or reach the Doylesville Church, you have gone too far. Please do not block traffic.

Intermediate access can be found at the park and surf where Cane Springs Road crosses the creek. From the intersection of College Hill Road (KY 977) and Oakley Wells Road, continue north on KY 977 to Cane Springs Road, at the Cane Springs Primitive Baptist Church. Turn left down the hill to the creek crossing.

Muddy Creek

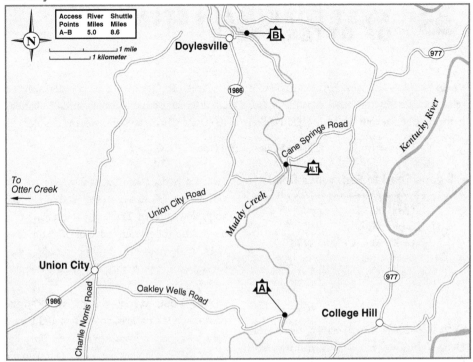

Access Points	River Miles	Shuttle Miles
A–B	5.0	8.6

⟡ **GAUGE** Check the Cane Springs Road Bridge. Look for the word "suck" painted by a vandal on the upstream bridge support. If the water is within 12 inches of "suck," then the creek is a runnable level.

GPS Coordinates

ACCESS	LATITUDE	LONGITUDE
A	N37° 47.292'	W84° 8.892'
B	N37° 50.741'	W84° 9.476'

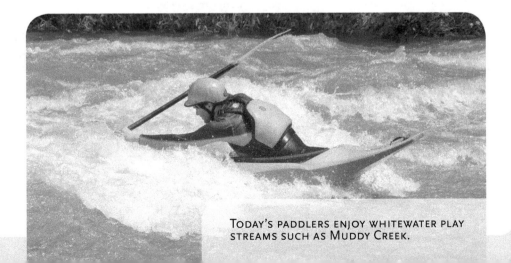

TODAY'S PADDLERS ENJOY WHITEWATER PLAY STREAMS SUCH AS MUDDY CREEK.

33 WEST FORK/MAIN STEM OF OTTER CREEK

◇ **OVERVIEW** The West Fork/Main Stem of Otter Creek provides quality whitewater with few difficulties for novice or skilled paddlers. It is a short distance from the put-in on Bill Eads Road to the confluence with the Main (Middle) Stem of the Otter, where the water volume doubles.

◇ **MAPS** RICHMOND NORTH (USGS)

Bill Eads Road to Sam Jones Road

Class	II (III)
Gauge	Visual
Level	Min. N/A–Max. N/A
Gradient	22.6'
Scenery	B

◇ **DESCRIPTION** The West Fork and Main Stem of the Otter is a very playful watershed littered with great surfing spots throughout its entire length. Easy, wide-open Class II rapids and the occasional Class III hydraulic prove Otter Creek to be another example of Madison County's wonderful whitewater bounty. Higher levels on the Otter will produce plenty of beautiful, large, smooth, and glassy surfing waves, as well as several large, sticky hydraulics easily boat scouted and avoided or surfed by skilled intermediate whitewater paddlers.

There are several alternate take-outs along its run to the Kentucky River, including the KY 3377 (Lost Fork Road) bridge, the confluence of the East Fork at KY 388, Sam Jones Road, and the KY 388 bridge close to Fort Boonesborough State Park (D).

◇ **SHUTTLE** The take-out is reached by continuing downstream on KY 388 from Red House to where a small paved road directly beside a house, Sam Jones Road, leaves KY 388 on the left down a steep hill at a sharp angle downstream. The take-out is just beyond the uncontrolled railroad crossing, on river right, underneath the bridge crossing Otter Creek. Do not go across the bridge; this is a private drive.

The standard put-in for Otter can be reached by taking Exit 90 on I-75 and taking the US 421/US 25 Bypass to KY 1986. Turn left on KY 1986 and follow it a short distance to KY 388, Red House Road. Follow KY 388 to Red House. Turn left off KY 388 at the Red House Church, onto Bill Eads Road. Drive several hundred yards upstream on river left and park at a turn-out on your left where Bill Eads turns right, away from the creek. Please park so as not to block the gravel access road to a field.

◇ **GAUGE** Check the bridge piling on KY 3377, Lost Fork Road. Zero inches is the minimum runnable level.

GPS COORDINATES

ACCESS	LATITUDE	LONGITUDE
A	N37° 50.738'	W84° 14.310'
B	N37° 50.735'	W84° 15.864'
C	N37° 52.272'	W84° 16.750'

West Fork/Main Stem of Otter Creek

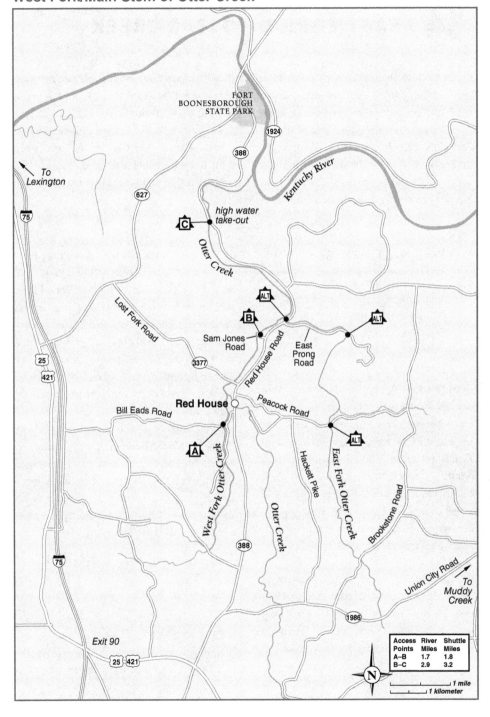

34 EAST FORK OF OTTER CREEK

◇ **OVERVIEW** Beginning as a narrow, intimate Class II stream, the East Fork of the Otter soon joins up with a small tributary just upstream of the bridge at East Prong Road. From this point, the creek then rushes swiftly through several significant Class III drops (IVs at high water) to the confluence at the Main Stem of the Otter. With a drainage area of only 15 miles, the East Fork of the Otter comes up and down very fast. Due to its relatively short length, it is usually run in tandem with the Main Stem of Otter Creek past the KY 388 (Red House Road) bridge, offering an additional 2–3 miles of Class II–III whitewater. Note that there is another Otter Creek in Meade County that flows directly into the Ohio River.

◇ **MAPS** Richmond North (USGS)

East Prong Road to KY 388

Class	II–III (IV)
Gauge	Visual
Level	Min. N/A–Max. N/A
Gradient	35.7'
Scenery	B

◇ **DESCRIPTION** The East Fork has continuous whitewater with numerous play possibilities, interesting broken limestone shelf drops, and some of the steepest gradients in central Kentucky. Hazards along the East Fork include deadfalls, sticky hydraulics at higher water levels, low clearance under a driveway bridge, and a second low-head dam-style driveway. Both driveways should be scouted from East Prong Road when water levels are very high.

◇ **SHUTTLE** There are two alternative put-ins on the East Fork. To gain the most creek mileage, take Peacock Road east from its intersection with KY 388 just north of the old Red House Grocery. Follow Peacock Road until it crosses the East Fork of the Otter. Put in at the bridge, taking care not to block the road. For the most popular shuttle used to run only the steepest section of the East Fork, take KY 388 to East Prong Road about 3 miles north of the old Red House Grocery. East Prong Road follows the East Fork of the Otter until it dead-ends at the bridge across the East Fork. Please park on the river left side of the bridge, because the river right side is private land. There are two main take-outs (although other possibilities exist). Use the KY 388 bridge across the East Fork of the Otter. This makes for the shortest run of the East Fork of the Otter and is typically used at low to moderate flow levels when runs on other Madison County streams are planned. Or use the KY 388 bridge across the Main Otter near Boonesborough State Park. This is usually the preferred take-out when water levels are very high. Use of this take-out allows for several miles of the Main Otter to be run in conjunction with the East Fork.

◇ **GAUGE** The only way to gauge this creek is to look at it.

GPS Coordinates

ACCESS	LATITUDE	LONGITUDE
A	N37° 49.518'	W84° 14.625'
B	N37° 50.745'	W84° 14.313'
C	N37° 50.929'	W84° 15.400'
D	N37° 52.272'	W84° 16.750'

East Fork of Otter Creek

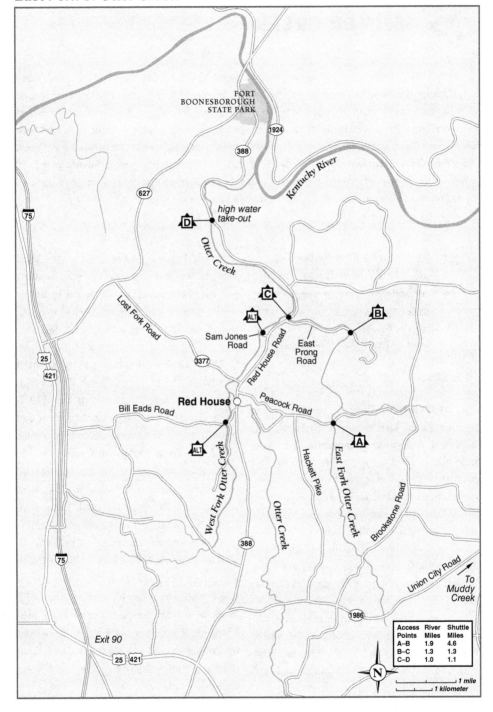

FORT BOONESBOROUGH STATE PARK

Kentucky River

high water take-out

Otter Creek

Lost Fork Road

Sam Jones Road

Red House Road

East Prong Road

Red House

Peacock Road

Bill Eads Road

West Fork Otter Creek

Hackett Pike

Otter Creek

East Fork Otter Creek

Brookstone Road

Union City Road

To Muddy Creek

Exit 90

Access Points	River Miles	Shuttle Miles
A–B	1.9	4.6
B–C	1.3	1.3
C–D	1.0	1.1

1 mile
1 kilometer

N

35   SILVER CREEK

✧ **OVERVIEW** Silver Creek boasts the largest watershed (112 square miles) of all of the Madison County whitewater streams and therefore will be most likely to hold its flow after a good rain. When doing a whitewater paddling Tour de Madison following a deluge rainfall, it is best to hold off on Silver Creek until the last and check out the other nearby streams first. East Fork Otter, Main Otter, Muddy, and Tates will all rise and drop at much faster rates than Silver Creek. After a moderate rain, when most of the others may not be running, look to Silver Creek first. Silver Creek consists of two main sections, allowing paddlers several options, ranging from an all-day tour to a short, no-shuttle-needed, play-filled half mile.

✧ **MAPS** KIRKSVILLE, RICHMOND SOUTH (USGS)

A   Curtis Pike Bridge to KY 876 Bridge

Class	I–III (IV)
Gauge	Visual
Level	Min. 0"; Opt. 1–2'–Max. 4'
Gradient	25'
Scenery	A

35A DESCRIPTION Silver Creek runs through scenic lush forest, beautiful rolling hills, and well-groomed farmland. The half mile above the KY 876 bridge features the popular park and surf section that contains several surfing spots and rapids, including Silver Creek Falls, which can be easily scouted from KY 876 just upstream of the bridge.

At optimum flows of 0 inches to 2 feet, Silver Creek is littered with numerous playful hydraulics among mostly Class II+ limestone ledge drops plus a scenic and runnable 4-foot river-wide ledge, locally known as Silver Creek Falls. At higher flows of 2–3 feet, Silver Creek approaches Class III through its short park and surf section. When gauge readings are 4 feet and higher, the swift, pushy water produces huge waves, increased possibility of large floating tree strainers and logjams, plus a significant but punchable recirculating hydraulic forming in the ledge of the third rapid in the park and surf section. Running just left of center and punching the hydraulic with strong momentum will help avoid getting caught in the very sticky right side.

✧ **SHUTTLE** The standard put-in is on a tributary of Silver Creek, Taylor Fork, which drains a fishing impoundment called Wilgreen Lake. The put-in is reached from Exit 87 on I-75 by heading west on KY 876, Barnes Mill Road. From Barnes Mill, turn left onto Curtis Pike and follow it to a small paved road that leads to the dam at Wilgreen Lake. Turn left and park alongside the road. Taylor Fork lies in the woods across Curtis Pike. If Taylor Fork is too low, continue on Curtis Pike to where a concrete bridge crosses Silver Creek and put in there. To reach the take-out from Exit 87 on I-75, take KY 876, Barnes Mill Road, west from the interstate to Bogie Mill Road, which continues straight on river right where Barnes Mill crosses Silver Creek from right to left on a concrete bridge, just beyond the Silver Creek Falls.

✧ **GAUGE** Check the visual gauge on KY 876 bridge over Silver Creek.

Silver Creek

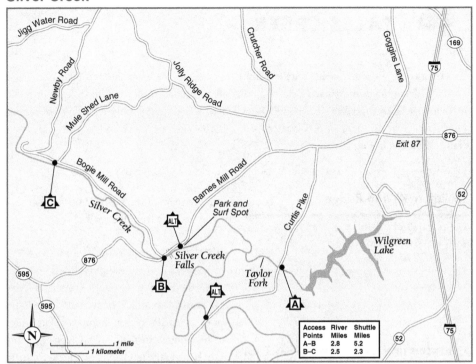

Access Points	River Miles	Shuttle Miles
A–B	2.8	5.2
B–C	2.5	2.3

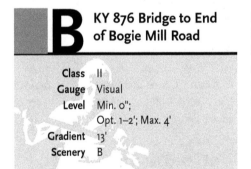

B KY 876 Bridge to End of Bogie Mill Road

Class II
Gauge Visual
Level Min. 0";
Opt. 1–2'; Max. 4'
Gradient 13'
Scenery B

35B DESCRIPTION The creek continues to be scenic, with herons and other bird species present along the way. The drops are not as frequent or steep as on the upper section.

SHUTTLE From Exit 87 on I-75, take KY 876, Barnes Mill Road, west from the interstate to Bogie Mill Road, which continues straight on river right, where Barnes Mill crosses Silver Creek from right to left on a concrete bridge, just beyond the Silver Creek

Falls. Follow Bogie Mill along the creek for about 2 miles, and continue on past Eddington Lane to where a low-water ford crosses over to farmland. Park take-out vehicles near the ford, making sure not to block access to it, though at high water levels the ford would obviously be impossible. The put-in is on Barnes Mill just before it crosses Silver Creek on the aforementioned concrete bridge.

GAUGE Check the visual gauge on the KY 876 bridge over Silver Creek.

GPS COORDINATES

ACCESS	LATITUDE	LONGITUDE
A	N37° 42.469'	W84° 21.825'
B	N37° 50.745'	W84° 14.313'
C	N37° 43.834'	W84° 25.652'

36 TATES CREEK

◇ **OVERVIEW** With one of the smallest drainage areas in Madison County, Tates Creek will crest and fall quickly and should be among one of the first a paddler should look for immediately following torrential rains. Though Tates typically is runnable only for a few hours, this creek is well worth the avid play boater's time. If you like fast water and big, playable wave trains, then this is your stream.

◇ **MAPS** RICHMOND NORTH, VALLEY VIEW (USGS)

Million to KY 169 Bridge

Class	II–III
Gauge	Visual
Level	Min. N/A–Max. N/A (cfs)
Gradient	30'
Scenery	B

◇ **DESCRIPTION** Tates Creek is one of the most accessible of Madison County's creeks, as it flows completely alongside KY 169, Tates Creek Road, just a few miles from I-75 and Richmond, Kentucky. This stream is essentially a continuous series of nonstop Class II–III surfing waves and holes with very few flat sections or defined drops. At high water levels, the flow is a fast, pushy freight train, producing huge waves that form up into groups in the steeper, narrower sections. Tates does not tend to wash out at flood levels, and higher water only means larger, more defined waves, holes, and fun for competent whitewater paddlers. Hazards along Tates Creek include strainers, especially along the section just upstream of the KY 1985 bridge that cannot be scouted from the road.

◇ **SHUTTLE** To reach the take-out from Exit 90 on I-75 south of Lexington, briefly take US 25 North, then turn left onto Keeneland Drive and travel 0.9 mile. Turn right onto Tates Creek Road/KY 169 and follow it 9.5 miles to the bridge crossing Tates Creek from the right bank to the left bank and the take-out. To reach the put-in from the take-out, backtrack on Tates Creek Road for 4.9 miles and turn right onto Maple Grove Road/KY 1984 and the bridge over Tates Creek.

◇ **GAUGE** Check the water level at the Million Church—if it is over the road, you are on your own.

GPS COORDINATES

ACCESS	LATITUDE	LONGITUDE
A	N37° 49.919'	W84° 25.114'
B	N37° 49.924'	W84° 25.127'

Tates Creek

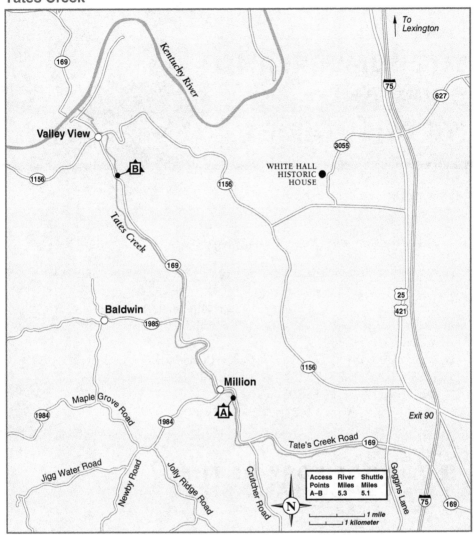

PART FIVE
THE CUMBERLAND RIVER AND ITS TRIBUTARIES

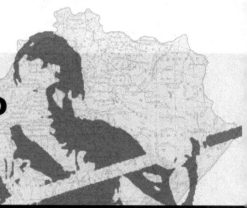

THE CUMBERLAND RIVER AND ITS TRIBUTARIES

37 POOR FORK OF THE CUMBERLAND RIVER

✧ **OVERVIEW** The Poor Fork of the Cumberland River drains Harlan and Letcher Counties in southeastern Kentucky and is the largest of the headwater streams of the North Fork of the Cumberland River. Flowing swiftly over a bed of rock and gravel, the Poor Fork winds through one of the deepest and most intimate mountain valleys in eastern Kentucky. Human habitation is frequently in evidence along the Poor Fork but does surprisingly little to spoil the incredible beauty of this mountain stream. Access is excellent due to US 119 passing through the valley, which crosses the Poor Fork many times.

✧ **MAPS** LOUELLEN, NOLANSBURG, EVARTS, HARLAN (USGS)

Poor Fork of the Cumberland River

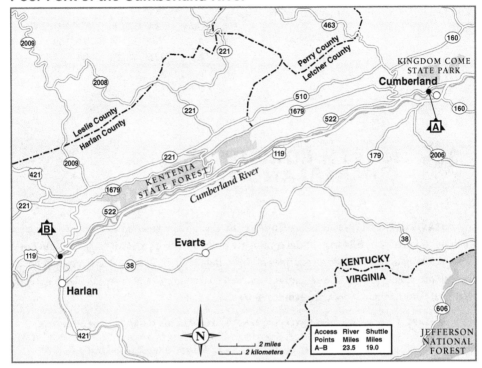

Cumberland to Harlan

Class	I–II
Gauge	Web
Level	Min. 4.5'–Max. flood
Gradient	10'
Scenery	B+

◇ **DESCRIPTION** Trees envelop the stream only intermittently, allowing paddlers frequent panoramic views of the surrounding mountains with luxurious foliage and exposed rock bluffs. The banks are normally 4–8 feet high and gently banked. The river varies in width from 25 to 40 feet and curves leisurely through the valley. Paddling is interesting, with continually changing vistas and delightful Class I and II small shoals and rapids. The Poor Fork is runnable from January through mid-April, and occasionally following heavy rains. Lateral erosion is minimal on the Poor Fork, so deadfalls are unusual. The only navigational hazards usually encountered are man-made concrete fords that cross the stream from time to time. Trips of nearly any distance are possible with the seemingly innumerable bridges over the Cumberland River on US 119. Beware the remains of a collapsed dam near the take-out in Harlan.

◇ **SHUTTLE** The take-out is located off KY 72 in Harlan, near the Arby's at the confluence of the Poor Fork Cumberland and Martins Fork. To reach the put-in from the take-out, follow US 119 North 21 miles to Cumberland, Kentucky. Turn left onto Frazier Street, then right onto Main Street and follow it 0.3 mile to turn left into the park located on the river near 408 Main Street.

✧ **GAUGE** The USGS gauge is Poor Fork at Cumberland, KY. Minimum reading should be 4.5 feet.

38 NORTH FORK OF THE CUMBERLAND RIVER

✧ **OVERVIEW** The North Fork of the Cumberland River (often referred to as simply the Cumberland) originates near Harlan at the confluence of the Poor Fork and Martins Fork and flows west, draining the east Kentucky counties of Knox, Bell, Harlan, Whitley, McCreary, and Pulaski. The run changes from Class I+ amid populated coal country, then enters the Daniel Boone National Forest, where the water becomes more challenging.

✧ **MAPS** HARLAN, WALLINS CREEK, BALKAN, VARILLA, MIDDLESBORO NORTH, PINEVILLE, ARTEMUS, BARBOURVILLE, ROCKHOLDS, SAXTON, WILLIAMSBURG, WOFFORD, CUMBERLAND FALLS, SAWYER (USGS); DANIEL BOONE NATIONAL FOREST MAP, SOUTH SECTION

A Harlan to West of Pineville

Class	I+
Gauge	Web
Level	Min. 300–Max. flood (cfs)
Gradient	2.5'
Scenery	C

38A **DESCRIPTION** To paddle the upper Cumberland is to become intimately acquainted with the land and the people of eastern Kentucky—their lifestyle and institutions are visible and alive all along the river. Although only steep, wooded hillsides meet your searching eyes, you are never out of earshot of the rumbling coal trucks or the raspy barking of a dog defending an unseen cabin in some lonely hollow.

Between Harlan and Pineville, the North Fork flows over a mud and gravel bed with infrequent small shoals and rapids (Class I+) and occasional large rocks in evidence in the stream and along the banks. From a width of approximately 50 feet at its origin, the Cumberland broadens quickly to 85–105 feet. Running west through the steep, rugged hills of the Cumberland Plateau, the river winds through forest and coal country, under hanging wooden footbridges, and past the cabins of miners and the ever-present coal tipples along the railroad tracks. The Cumberland from Harlan to Pineville is frequently runnable from November through mid-May. Access is reasonably good, providing you are accustomed to steep banks.

North Fork of the Cumberland River: Harlan to West of Pineville

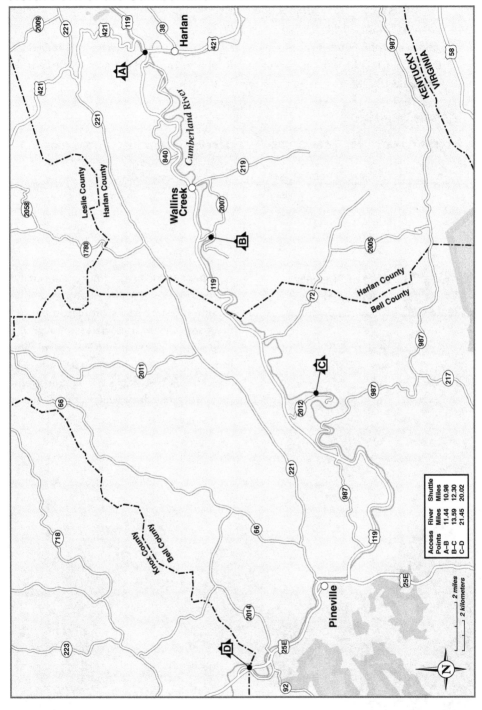

Access Points	River Miles	Shuttle Miles
A–B	11.44	10.98
B–C	13.59	12.30
C–D	21.45	20.02

⟡ SHUTTLE To reach the take-out from Pineville, take US 25E north for 3.2 miles, then turn right onto KY 2014 and follow it 0.1 mile to the bridge over the Cumberland River. To reach the put-in from the take-out, backtrack to Pineville and take US 119 for 35 miles to Harlan. Turn right onto US 421, then immediately turn right again onto KY 72 to reach the bridge over the Cumberland.

⟡ GAUGE The USGS gauge is Cumberland River near Harlan. Minimum reading should be 300 cfs.

GPS Coordinates

ACCESS	LATITUDE	LONGITUDE	ACCESS	LATITUDE	LONGITUDE
A	N36° 51.669'	W83° 19.505'	C	N36° 45.862'	W83° 33.788'
B	N36° 49.418'	W83° 27.264'	D	N36° 48.063'	W83° 45.296'

B West of Pineville to Williamsburg

Class	I+
Gauge	Web
Level	Min. 300–Max. flood (cfs)
Gradient	2.5'
Scenery	C+

38B DESCRIPTION As the Cumberland passes Pineville, it settles down into a mud bottom with steep banks, broadens a bit, and flows smoothly as it progresses through the deep valleys past Barbourville toward Williamsburg. The section from Harlan to Williamsburg is best suited to 1-day runs (pick your own) rather than paddle camping. Access

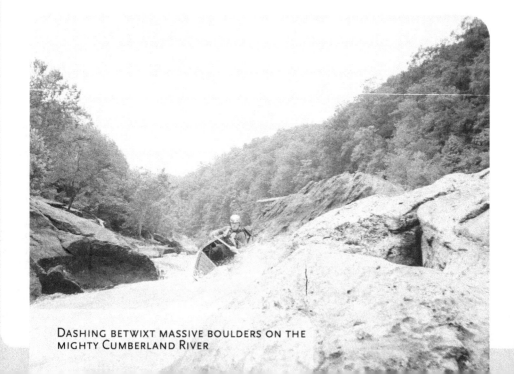

DASHING BETWIXT MASSIVE BOULDERS ON THE MIGHTY CUMBERLAND RIVER

North Fork of the Cumberland River:
West of Pineville to Williamsburg

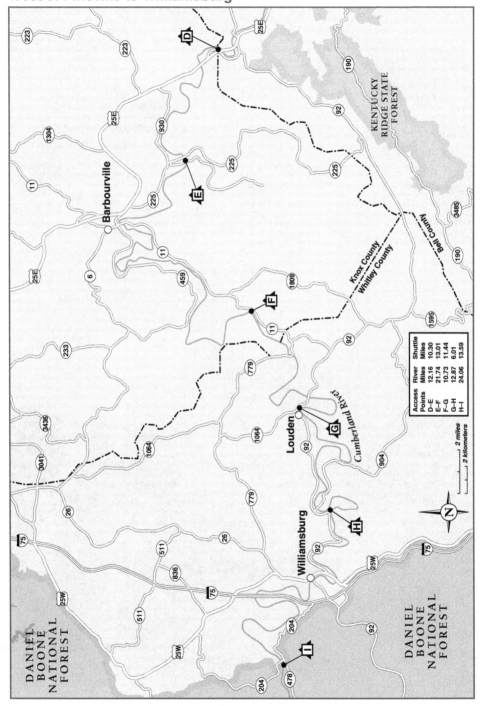

Access Points	River Miles	Shuttle Miles
D–E	12.16	10.30
E–F	21.74	13.01
F–G	10.73	11.44
G–H	12.87	6.01
H–I	24.06	13.59

points between Pineville and Williamsburg are numerous, as many bridges cross the river and allow trips of varied lengths. It is 34 miles from the put-in west of Pineville to the KY 1530 bridge, 11 miles from the KY 1530 bridge to the KY 92 bridge, and 37 miles to the boat ramp downstream of the Red Bird Bridge, just west of Williamsburg.

✧ **SHUTTLE** To reach the take-out from Williamsburg, take KY 204 North/Red Bird Road 4.6 miles to meet KY 478. Stay straight on KY 478 and follow it 0.3 mile to the boat ramp on your right. To reach the put-in from the take-out, backtrack to Williamsburg and take KY 92 East 34 miles. Turn left onto KY 2014 and

travel 0.6 mile to reach the bridge over the Cumberland River.

✧ **GAUGE** The USGS gauge is Cumberland River near Harlan. Minimum reading should be 300 cfs.

GPS Coordinates

ACCESS	LATITUDE	LONGITUDE
D	N36° 48.063'	W83° 45.296'
E	N36° 49.346'	W83° 50.395'
F	N36° 46.880'	W83° 57.195'
G	N36° 45.081'	W84° 1.701'
H	N36° 43.926'	W84° 6.258'
I	N36° 45.718'	W84° 13.334'

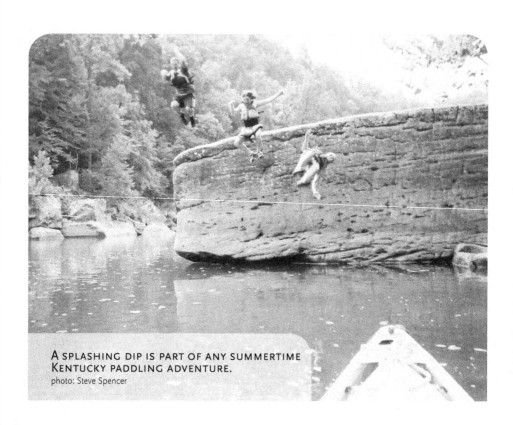

A SPLASHING DIP IS PART OF ANY SUMMERTIME KENTUCKY PADDLING ADVENTURE.
photo: Steve Spencer

C Williamsburg to Cumberland Falls

Class	II
Gauge	Web
Level	Min. 400–Max. 2,000/flood open/decked (cfs)
Gradient	2.6'
Scenery	B

38C DESCRIPTION From Williamsburg to Cumberland Falls, the river flows through the Daniel Boone National Forest. Access for this section is not plentiful but is good where it exists. The boat ramp below the Red Bird Bridge makes for a fine access (I). The Cumberland from Williamsburg to Cumberland Falls is normally runnable from November to early June.

In this section, the river continues to widen until in some places it is almost 200 feet across. The gradient increases here also and some mild whitewater (Class II) is encountered, with boulders in the stream and some shoals spanning the entire width of the river. This section (beyond the mouth of Jellico Creek) is extremely remote and makes a good paddle-camping run at moderate water levels (500–1,100 cfs) and a fair whitewater run at higher levels (1,100–1,900 cfs). Rock replaces the mud bottom of the upper sections, and the current runs swift and continuously with very few pools. Boulders line the banks in increasing numbers, and some flat, accessible terraces have been carved along the streamside.

North Fork of the Cumberland River: Williamsburg to Cumberland Falls

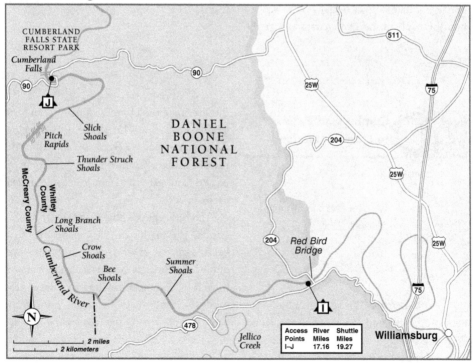

In the last 3 miles before reaching the KY 90 bridge, exposed rock palisades become visible on the right as the Cumberland begins to enter the deep gorge that will carry it over the falls and beyond to Lake Cumberland.

About 1 mile upstream of the falls, the river curves sharply to the left, and the KY 90 bridge becomes visible downstream. Move to the right of the river for the take-out on the upstream side of the bridge (at the picnic ground and parking lot). Failure to move promptly to the right can have tragic consequences for the unlucky or inexperienced. One of the larger shoals (Class II) of this section is situated across the entire river just upstream of the take-out. If you run it on the left and fill up or capsize, you will find yourself in the main current heading for the entrance rapids to Cumberland Falls several hundred yards downstream. If you run the shoals on the right and take water or turn over, you will be in much slower current and (except at excessive levels, that is, 1,900+ cfs) will be washed into the bank as the river narrows near the

bridge, or alternately swept downstream past the bridge into a huge eddy that forms along the bank near the visitors' parking lot.

✧ **SHUTTLE** From Exit 15 on I-75 take US 25W North to KY 90. Turn left and take KY 90 West to Cumberland Falls State Park. To reach the put-in, return to US 25W via KY 90 and head south on 25W to KY 204. Turn right and take KY 204 South to the Redbird Bridge over the Cumberland. Once across the bridge turn right onto KY 478 and follow it a short distance to the boat ramp on your right.

✧ **GAUGE** The USGS gauge is Cumberland River at Williamsburg. A flow of 400 cfs is minimum, and 3,000 cfs is the upper runnable limit.

GPS Coordinates

ACCESS	LATITUDE	LONGITUDE
I	N36° 45.718'	W84° 13.334'
J	N36° 50.181'	W84° 20.547'

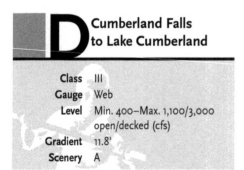

Cumberland Falls to Lake Cumberland

Class	III
Gauge	Web
Level	Min. 400–Max. 1,100/3,000 open/decked (cfs)
Gradient	11.8'
Scenery	A

38D **DESCRIPTION** This section of the North Fork of Cumberland is a Kentucky-protected Wild River and is one of the most popular whitewater runs in the state. Referred to as the Cumberland below the Falls by local paddlers,

the river here runs through a mammoth rock gorge with boulders lining the river marking the age-old headward erosion of the falls. The run should be attempted only by experienced boaters, and extra flotation is recommended for open boats.

The run begins with a long carry from the visitors' parking lot at Cumberland Falls to a beach a quarter of a mile away at the bottom of the falls. Scenery is spectacular right from the put-in, and most paddlers take the opportunity to paddle back upstream for a truly awe-inspiring view of the falls (80 yards from the falls is as close as you can safely paddle without fighting a fantastically strong reversal current seeking to pull you into the falls).

North Fork of the Cumberland River:
Cumberland Falls to Lake Cumberland

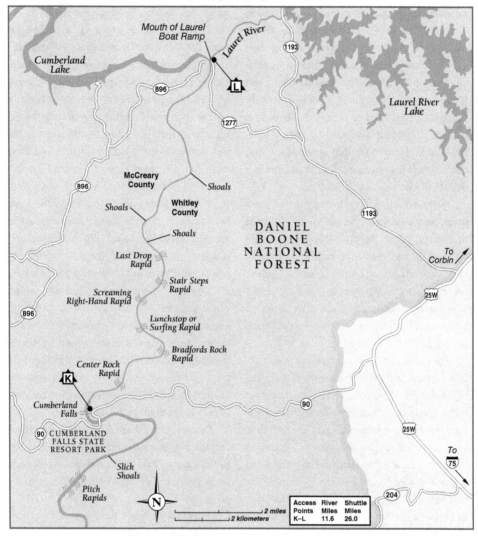

Moving downstream, several easy Class II rapids that require no scouting are encountered before arriving at the Class III Center Rock Rapid. This rapid can be identified by the large boulders on each side that constrict the river to a channel of approximately 20 feet, and by the degree of drop that substantially exceeds that encountered previously. The rapid consists of a 25-foot-long, stair-step chute followed 50 feet later by a 3-foot vertical drop directly in front of a huge boulder that splits the current. This is Center Rock. The first drop is usually run straight down the center, and the strategy for the second is to angle the bow to the right and drop straight into the eddy on the right at the bottom of the drop. An alternate strategy for the second drop is to ride the pillow off the right side of Center Rock. It is recommended that this rapid be scouted.

Continuing downstream, the river lapses into a series of pools followed by rock gardens (at low to moderate water) and Class II rapids. The drops are small, but several of the rapids are quite technical. One of these, at about mile 4, has an undercut boulder situated in mid-channel, splitting the flow. This should be run along the far right bank. Moving on, there are more long pools and small rapids. At mile 5, there is a slanting 2.5-foot drop with a playful hole at the bottom that spans the entire river. This is known as Surfing Rapid and is a delightful place to stop for lunch.

Beyond Surfing Rapid, the run becomes more intense. One-half mile downstream of Surfing Rapid, the river disappears to the right around a house-size rock and immediately cuts left again, crashing into a boulder on the right and down a 30-foot-long chute. This intense, borderline Class III run serves up an exciting ride. Run right center and play the pillow off the boulder.

The next rapid, a quarter mile distant, is a turning 4-foot drop known as Screaming Right-Hand Rapid. At low to moderate water levels the main flow drops over a 1.5-foot ledge and splashes almost immediately on a rock that diverts the current sharply to the right over a 3-foot slanted drop. The most popular strategy here is to cut right after the first ledge, using the pillow to turn the boat. At higher water levels, the river overflows the obstructing rock and a 4-foot vertical drop and a mean hydraulic is created completely across the river. Scouting is definitely required in this situation. Screaming Right-Hand Rapid becomes Class IV at higher water levels.

The next large rapid, known as Stair Steps, is a long, delightful, borderline Class III stretch that looks much worse than it is. It is easily recognized by the large hole at the top with a shark fin–shaped rock just below it. Decked boaters may want to punch the hole.

For open boaters, the best route is to run right of the hole and then hug the right bank all the way to the bottom. Scout on the right.

The last major rapid is appropriately named Last Drop. In this Class III area, the current winds to the right along the upstream side of a large boulder and then suddenly cuts left, dropping vertically 3 feet. Next, the current is split by a building-size boulder in the middle of the river. Run to the right at the top, staying to the inside of the turn and away from the upstream face of the boulder. Cut hard left, taking the vertical drop as close to the boulder as possible. Go around the huge boulder that splits the current on the far right. At high water, this rapid (like several others) changes drastically, forming a supermean hole at the top. Scout (or portage) to the right.

Last Drop marks the end of the whitewater section of the Cumberland (although several small shoals are encountered farther downstream due to the low level of the lake pool). From here, it is a scenic 3.5-mile paddle through the lake to the take-out at the mouth of the Laurel River on Lake Cumberland. Access is excellent at the take-out.

Dangers other than those already described include logs that occasionally become trapped in the narrower chutes and strong headwinds while paddling off the lake.

◇ **SHUTTLE** To reach the take-out from Exit 25 on I-75 near Corbin, take US 25W south 4.7 miles. Turn right onto KY 1193 North and follow it 4.6 miles to reach Bee Creek Road/CR 1277. Keep straight on Bee Creek Road and go 3.3 miles to Mouth of Laurel boat ramp on Laurel River Lake. To reach the put-in from the take-out, backtrack to US 25W and turn right, heading south for 2.5 miles. Turn right onto KY 90 West and go a little over 7 miles to Cumberland Falls State Park and the beach access below the falls.

✧ **GAUGE** The USGS gauge is Cumberland River at Williamsburg. A flow of 400 cfs is minimum, and 3,000 cfs is the upper runnable limit.

GPS Coordinates

ACCESS	LATITUDE	LONGITUDE
K	N36° 50.336'	W84° 20.645'
L	N36° 56.718'	W84° 17.743'

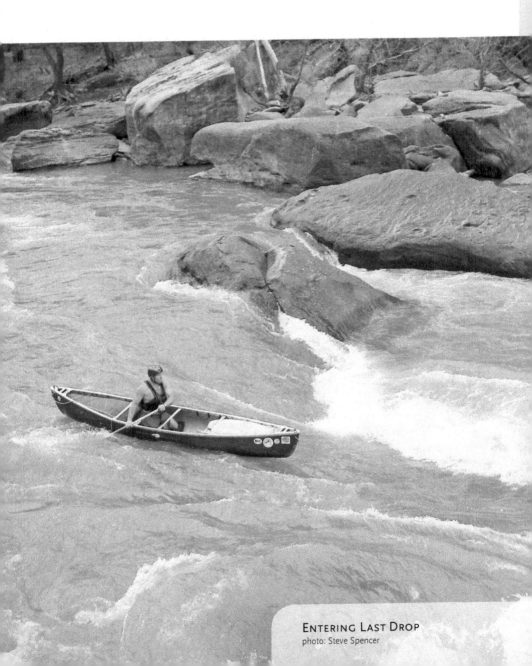

ENTERING LAST DROP
photo: Steve Spencer

39 **LAUREL RIVER**

◇ **OVERVIEW** Spectacular scenery, great rapids, but tough to catch in its entirety at runnable levels characterizes this 2-mile remnant of the Laurel River. The flow in this stretch below the U.S. Army Corps of Engineers' Laurel River Dam is controlled by the East Kentucky Power Cooperative of Winchester (EKP), whose erratic releases can provide about 2 miles of fun rapids in very cold water.

◇ **MAPS** DANIEL BOONE NATIONAL FOREST, SOUTH SECTION

Laurel River Dam to Lake Cumberland

Class	Class II–III (IV)
Gauge	Phone
Level	Min. N/A–Max. N/A
Gradient	30'
Scenery	A

◇ **DESCRIPTION** Predictions of releases are very difficult—even for EKP—as the dam is used to provide peak power electrical generation. Even at the height of the summer, paddlers will want to take along cold-weather boating gear, because the release water flows from the bottom of Laurel Lake and is ice cold. Though runnable year-round, the Laurel is

Laurel River

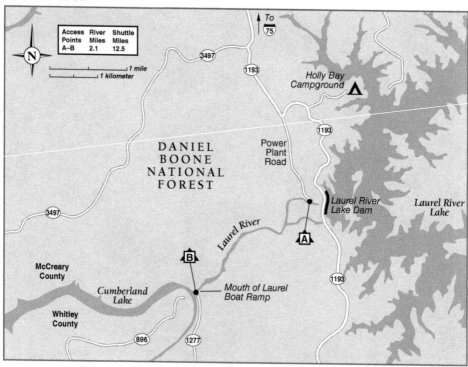

probably best caught in August and September, when hot temperatures increase the national demand for electrical power generation. Unfortunately, due to typical summer pool levels for Lake Cumberland, a summertime run on the Laurel could mean that the final and only Class IV rapid, Whorehouse, will be covered under the lake's stagnant flatwater.

✧ **SHUTTLE** To reach the take-out from Exit 25 on I-75 near Corbin, take US 25W south 4.7 miles. Turn right onto KY 1193 North and follow it 4.6 miles to reach Bee Creek Road/ CR 1277. Keep straight on Bee Creek Road for 3.3 miles to Mouth of Laurel boat ramp on Laurel River Lake. To reach the put-in from the take-out, backtrack to KY 1193, turn left, and follow it north for 5.2 miles. Turn left onto Forest Road 4005, then keep straight on Power Plant Road and follow it 1 mile to dead-end at the tailwater of the Laurel River.

✧ **GAUGE** Flow from the Laurel Lake Dam controlled by EKP in Winchester. Highly unpredictable. Call EKP at 859-744-4812 for flow report.

GPS Coordinates		
ACCESS	**LATITUDE**	**LONGITUDE**
A	N36° 57.710'	W84° 16.268'
B	N36° 56.718'	W84° 17.743'

40 ROCKCASTLE RIVER

✧ **OVERVIEW** The Rockcastle River, a Kentucky state Blue Water Trail, originates in Laurel County and drains portions of Jackson, Rockcastle, Laurel, and Pulaski Counties. One of Kentucky's most popular rivers, the Rockcastle offers something for every type of paddle, from Class I paddle camping to challenging Class III–IV kayaker whitewater. The scenery is appealing in this part of the Daniel Boone National Forest.

✧ **MAPS** LIVINGSTON, BERNSTADT, BILLOWS, ANO, SAWYER (USGS); DANIEL BOONE NATIONAL FOREST MAP, SOUTH SECTION

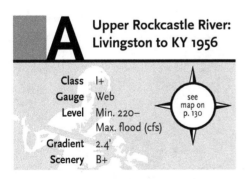

A Upper Rockcastle River: Livingston to KY 1956

Class	I+
Gauge	Web
Level	Min. 220–
	Max. flood (cfs)
Gradient	2.4'
Scenery	B+

see map on p. 130

sand and rock bed through hilly woods and farmland in the heart of the Daniel Boone National Forest. Runnable from late fall to midsummer, this section is scenic and has banks of varying steepness and some very mild (Class I+) whitewater. A favorite run for paddle campers, current is good and dangers to navigation are limited to deadfalls. An alternate access allowing a shorter day trip is under the I-75 bridge off KY 1329.

 DESCRIPTION The upper sections from KY 490 to KY 1956 (old KY 80), flow over a

✧ **SHUTTLE** To reach the take-out from Exit 49 on I-75, take KY 909 North to US 25. Turn

Upper Rockcastle River: Livingston to KY 1956

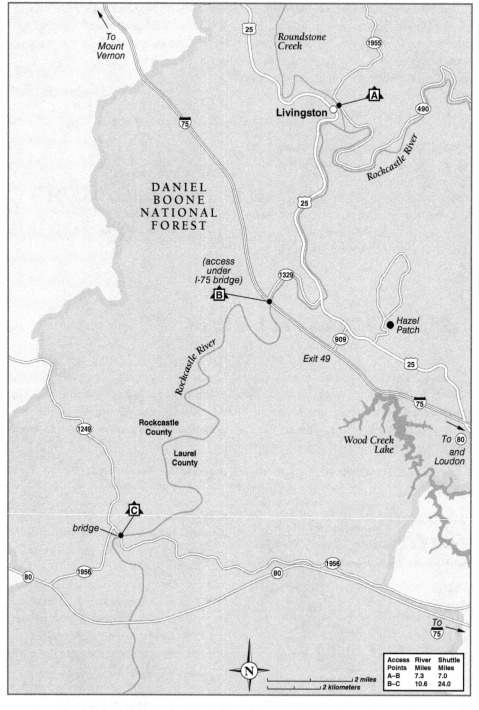

left onto US 25 North, then take another left turn onto KY 1329 and follow it to the access under the I-75 bridge. To reach the put-in from the take-out, backtrack to US 25, turn left, and follow it north to KY 490 East and the bridge over Rockcastle Creek in Livingston. Turn right just after the bridge to reach an access.

⟡ **GAUGE** The USGS gauge is Rockcastle River at Billows. Minimum reading should be 220 cfs.

GPS COORDINATES

ACCESS	LATITUDE	LONGITUDE
A	N37° 17.928'	W84° 12.804'
B	N37° 14.442'	W84° 14.378'

ACCESS	LATITUDE	LONGITUDE
C	N37° 10.272'	W84° 17.814'

≈≈≈

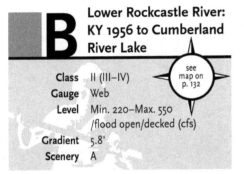

B Lower Rockcastle River: KY 1956 to Cumberland River Lake

see map on p. 132

Class	II (III–IV)
Gauge	Web
Level	Min. 220–Max. 550 /flood open/decked (cfs)
Gradient	5.8'
Scenery	A

40B **DESCRIPTION** The lower Rockcastle, from KY 1956 to KY 192, is a protected Kentucky Wild River and is one of Kentucky's most popular whitewater runs. The scenery is splendid, with tall, forested hills along the first miles of the run giving way to high rock bluffs further downstream, with boxcar-size boulders situated in the river and along the banks. Paddling the lower Rockcastle is both interesting and challenging. To begin with, the run used to be an exhausting 17 miles long. However, the old Howard Place offers a put-in that cuts off most of the upper Class I water that allows for runs only of the Beech Narrows.

The first 6 miles are essentially Class I with a fair current and numerous riffles and small ledges. Throughout the next 6 miles, the river picks up a little gradient and

several honest Class II rapids are encountered. Although these rapids are not difficult, two or three do disappear around boulders or curves. If you are not intimately familiar with the river (this or any other), you should take the time to scout these. Guidebook or no, it is not healthy to get into the habit of running rapids of which you cannot see the end. The Howard Place access is around mile 11. At about mile 12 the river curves hard right and then hard left, tumbling down a Class II (III?) series of ledges and standing waves known as the Stair Steps. Beyond this rapid, the Rockcastle reverts to long pools punctuated by short Class II drops at the ends.

At about mile 15, the river appears to come to a dead end in a large boulder garden, but closer inspection reveals that whole stream is grunting laboriously between two huge rocks and falling about 4 feet. This is Beech (Creek) Narrows. Above the drop, an ill-placed boulder makes it difficult to set up. Below the drop is a very bad, highly aerated keeper hydraulic. Beyond the hydraulic, the current washes directly into a large boulder. Though this Class IV rapid has been run both decked and open, we consider attempting to run it in an open boat very dangerous, with success more a function of luck (specifically, catching

Lower Rockcastle River: KY 1956 to Cumberland River Lake

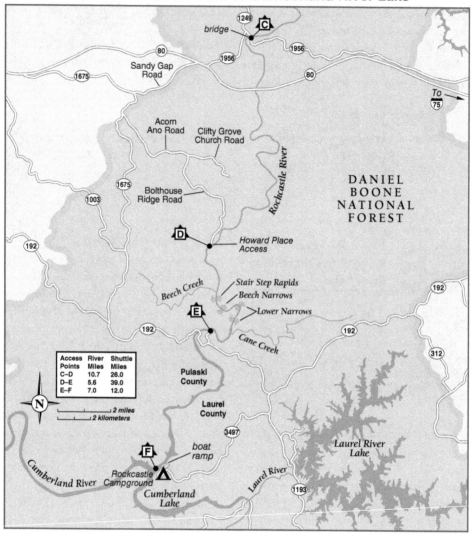

the rotation of the violent hydraulic on the up cycle, where it helps kick you free) than skill. A portage trail circles the boulders on the right. Our advice: carry around. If you choose to run, set up a rescue person where you are certain you can reach a person trapped in the keeper on the first throw.

Below Beech Narrows, the Rockcastle assumes its normal pool and drop for another three-quarters of a mile before entering a

second apparent cul-de-sac. Here the river forms a large, tranquil pool before cutting hard right, churning down a fast chute, and smacking into a rock. This rapid marks the entrance to the Lower Narrows, a three-quarter-mile stretch of intense and almost continuous, highly technical Class III and IV water. After the first rapid of the Lower Narrows (which is followed by a 200-yard pool), the remaining four rapids are lined up literally one behind the other in an amazing stretch of tumbling, turbulent whitewater that lambastes the paddler with every challenge in the book. There are, thankfully however, some large eddies that let an embattled paddler stop after each rapid to bail, collect wits, and scramble up the banks to scout whatever lurks ahead.

The rapids of the Lower Narrows are all runnable, but they demand considerable expertise in water reading and whitewater tactics. They also demand considerable time. The whole narrows is a series of twisting, turning, blind drops so that it is impossible to see what lies beyond the next ledge. Thus, each rapid must be scouted individually. This entails a seemingly endless routine of jumping in and out of boats and scrambling up immense boulders to sneak a look at the next rapid. The scouting and the boulder hopping

are necessary, of course, but also time consuming. A good running time for the Lower Narrows by an experienced group of four open-canoe tandem teams would be about 2 hours. The alternative to running the Narrows is carrying via a trail on the east bank that is reached by climbing the bank at the end of the pool marking the entrance to the first rapid. In running the Lower Rockcastle, time is always a prime consideration. Therefore, whitewater enthusiasts will want to start at Howard Place, running the Narrows at their leisure.

Beyond the Lower Narrows, there are a Class II and a borderline Class III stretch that are blind turns and should be scouted. The first rapid (the Class II) particularly has a tendency to trap floating logs in the spring. Downstream from the Class III it is approximately 1 mile to the take-out at Bee Rock Boat Ramp.

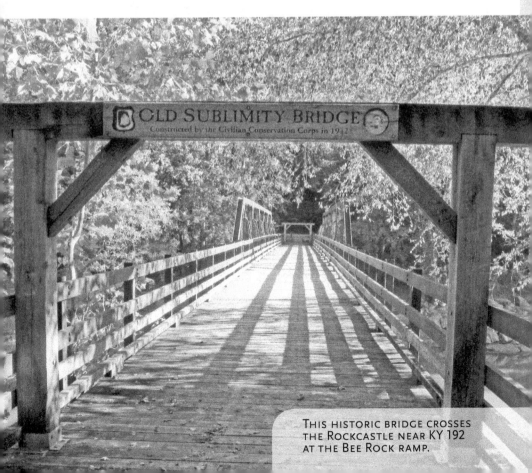

THIS HISTORIC BRIDGE CROSSES THE ROCKCASTLE NEAR KY 192 AT THE BEE ROCK RAMP.

As you might gather, the Rockcastle River is beautiful, challenging, and exhausting if this entire section is run in a single day. The paddler has more than put in a full day before even reaching the most demanding part of the run. An early put-in (10 a.m. at the absolute latest) is a necessity. Only paddlers with a lot of experience on technical rivers should attempt the Lower Narrows. Extra flotation is a must for open canoes. Dangers other than those already mentioned include deadfalls on several turns along the first 12 miles. Access is good at both put-in and take-out. Average stream width is 40–60 feet. A much calmer paddle can be enjoyed by all on Lake Cumberland, for 7 miles from Bee Rock to the Rockcastle Campground boat ramp off KY 1193.

✧ **SHUTTLE** To reach the take-out from Exit 38 on I-75 near London, head west on KY 192 18 miles to the bridge over the Rockcastle River. The Bee Rock Boat Ramp is on the east side of the river. To reach the put-in from Exit 41 on I-75, take KY 80 West to KY 1956. Turn right on KY 1956 and follow it west to bridge over Rockcastle on outfitter on left before river. To reach the Howard Place access from Exit 41 on I-75, take KY 80 West to Sandy Gap Road, on the west side of the KY 80 bridge over the Rockcastle. Turn left on Sandy Gap Road and follow it to KY 1675. Turn left onto KY 1675 and follow it to Acorn Ano Road. Turn left on Acorn Ano Road and follow it to Bolthouse Ridge Road. Turn right on Bolthouse Ridge Road, which passes through reclaimed strip-mine land. Follow Bolthouse Ridge Road as it descends to the Rockcastle and Lick Creek, about 2 miles above Beech Creek. A four-wheel-drive vehicle with high ground clearance is wise on the lower part of Bolthouse Road, especially after rains.

✧ **GAUGE** The USGS gauge is Rockcastle River at Billows. The minimum reading should be 220 cfs.

GPS Coordinates

ACCESS	LATITUDE	LONGITUDE
C	N37° 10.272'	W84° 17.814'
D	N37° 4.147'	W84° 19.354'
E	N37° 1.681'	W84° 19.320'
F	N36° 57.601'	W84° 21.303'

41 BUCK CREEK

✧ **OVERVIEW** Buck Creek is a small, scenic, Class II whitewater stream that drains the eastern half of Pulaski County. Several small caves along the run provide the opportunity for interesting side trips. Runnable from KY 1677 to KY 192 following periods of heavy rain, Buck Creek winds through forested hillsides with some exposed rock visible, especially in the lower sections below KY 80.

✧ **MAPS** SHOPVILLE, DYKES (USGS)

Buck Creek

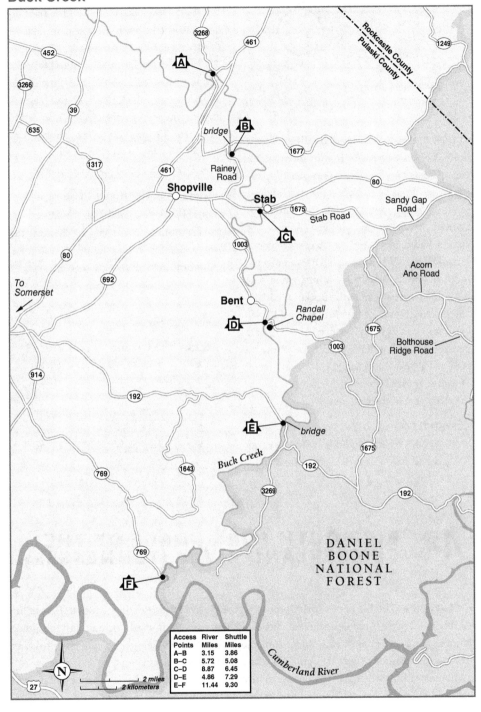

Access Points	River Miles	Shuttle Miles
A–B	3.15	3.86
B–C	5.72	5.08
C–D	8.87	6.45
D–E	4.86	7.29
E–F	11.44	9.30

KY 1677 to KY 192

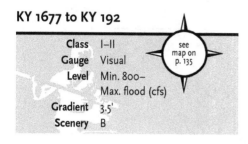

Class	I–II
Gauge	Visual
Level	Min. 800–
	Max. flood (cfs)
Gradient	3.5'
Scenery	B

see map on p. 135

◆ **DESCRIPTION** The level of difficulty on Buck Creek is easy Class II with most rapids consisting of very small ledges or small standing waves. Route selection is obvious, and no scouting is required. Deadfalls constitute the primary hazard to navigation. The average stream width is 35–45 feet. Access is good, including the KY 1003 bridge (D). Water levels on Buck Creek are usually optimal when surrounding larger streams (the Rockcastle River and the North Fork of the Cumberland River) are high or marginally flooded. The run can be extended below KY 192 to Lake Cumberland at KY 769 (F) (reached from Somerset). However, most of these final 11.5 miles are on the slack pool of the lake.

◆ **SHUTTLE** To reach the put-in from Somerset, take KY 80 East to KY 461. Turn left on KY 461 and follow it to KY 1677. Turn right on KY 1677 and follow it to Rainey Road, just before bridge over Buck Creek. Turn right on Rainey Road and reach an access on left. To reach access E from Somerset, take KY 80 East to KY 914. Turn right on KY 914 and follow it to KY 192. Turn left on KY 192 and travel east to the bridge over Buck Creek. To reach access F from downtown Somerset, take KY 80 east to turn right on KY 914. Take KY 914 south to turn left on KY 769. Stay with KY 769 all the way to the Buck Creek Ramp on Lake Cumberland.

◆ **GAUGE** Buck Creek is a look-and-see proposition. However, a good guesstimate can be made for running Buck Creek by checking the USGS gauge for Rockcastle River at Billows. The minimum reading should be 800 cfs.

GPS COORDINATES

ACCESS	LATITUDE	LONGITUDE
A	N37° 12.630'	W84° 27.882'
B	N37° 10.560'	W84° 27.290'
C	N37° 9.097'	W84° 26.329'
D	N37° 6.194'	W84° 26.181'
E	N37° 3.586'	W84° 25.612'
F	N36° 59.628'	W84° 29.668'

42 BIG SOUTH FORK GORGE OF THE CUMBERLAND RIVER (TENNESSEE)

◆ **OVERVIEW** The Big South Fork Gorge is part of the headwaters of the Big South Fork of the Cumberland River. Although situated entirely in Tennessee, it is worth including in this guide because it is a very popular whitewater run enjoyed by advanced Kentucky paddlers. Consisting of almost continuous Class III (and IV?) whitewater, the run begins on the Clear Fork (which combines with New River of Tennessee to form the Big South Fork of the Cumberland River) about 12 miles southwest of Oneida and ends at Leatherwood Ford, west of Oneida.

◆ **MAPS** ONEIDA SOUTH, HONEY CREEK (USGS); BIG SOUTH FORK NATIONAL RIVER AND RECREATION AREA MAP

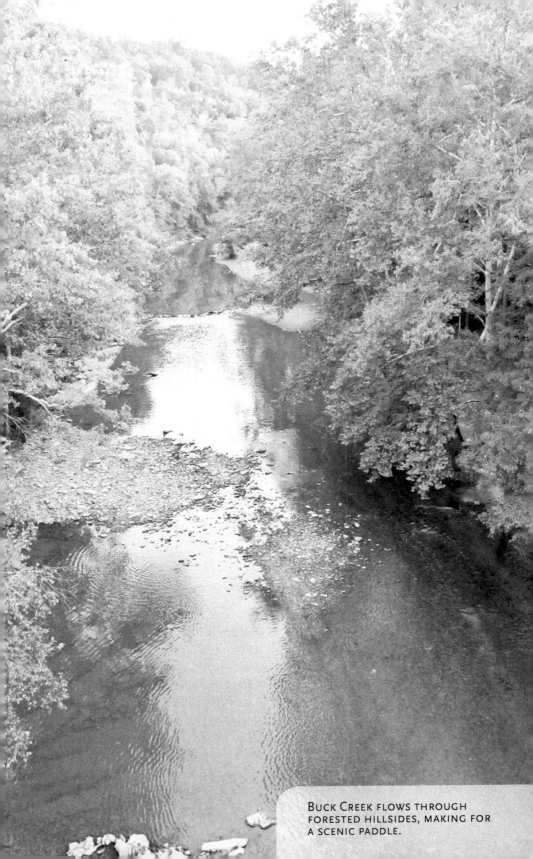

BUCK CREEK FLOWS THROUGH
FORESTED HILLSIDES, MAKING FOR
A SCENIC PADDLE.

Big South Fork Gorge of the Cumberland River (Tennessee)

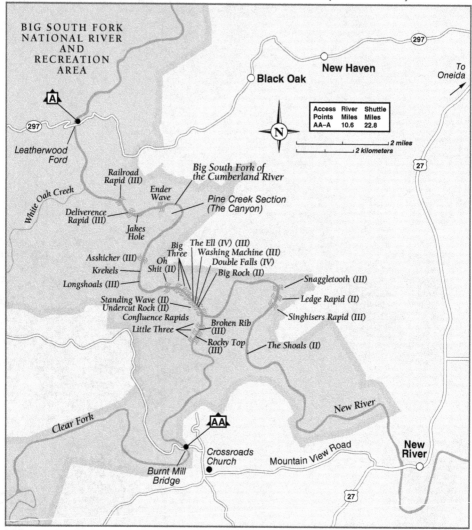

Burnt Mill Bridge to Leatherwood Ford

Class	III–IV
Gauge	Web
Level	Min. 450–Max. 6,000 (cfs)
Gradient	19.5'
Scenery	A+

✧ **DESCRIPTION** In all, there are 13 major rapids and several dozen smaller ones in the upper Big South Fork Gorge. Considered by

many to be a decked-boat and rafting river, the Big South Fork Gorge is run successfully on by both solo and tandem open-boaters, but primarily kayakers these days. The nature of the run varies incredibly with water level, being extremely technical at lower water and big and pushy (much like the New River Gorge in West Virginia) when flowing high. At moderate levels, paddlers get a taste of both worlds with quick, technical water on the Clear Fork and bigger, less technical water below the confluence (of the Clear Fork and the New River). Scenery is magnificent, when you have time to notice it, with boulders lining the banks and canyon walls rising on both sides. For a Class III (IV) river, the Big South Fork Gorge is mostly free of dangers; deadfalls and logjams are infrequent, and the holes are washouts at almost all levels. However, watch out for undercut rocks that have resulted in close calls in the past. The drops, however, are sizable (several exceeding 4 feet), and helmets are a must for all paddlers. Also, some of the rapids are extremely long, making rescue difficult (especially at higher water levels). Extra flotation is essential for open canoes, and a good roll is definitely recommended for decked boaters. Access at the river is good at both put-in and take-out, with large boater parking area. The Big South Fork Gorge is runnable from late fall to mid-May in years of average rainfall.

✧ **SHUTTLE** To access the take-out from Oneida, Tennessee, take TN 297 West 11 miles to Leatherwood Fork access on the right before the bridge over the Big South Fork. To reach the put-in from the take-out, return to Oneida and take US 27 South 10 miles. Turn right onto Old US 27 and go 1.4 miles; then turn right toward Mountain View Road and make a quick left to join Mountain View Road for 2.3 miles. Turn right onto Al Martin Road and follow it 0.5 mile. Turn left onto Honey Creek Loop Road and reach Burnt Mill Bridge paddler access after 0.4 mile.

✧ **GAUGE** The USGS gauge is South Fork Cumberland River at Leatherwood Ford, TN. The minimum level is 450 cfs; the maximum level is 6,000 cfs.

GPS Coordinates

ACCESS	LATITUDE	LONGITUDE
AA	N36° 23.257'	W84° 37.757'
A	N36° 28.637'	W84° 40.098'

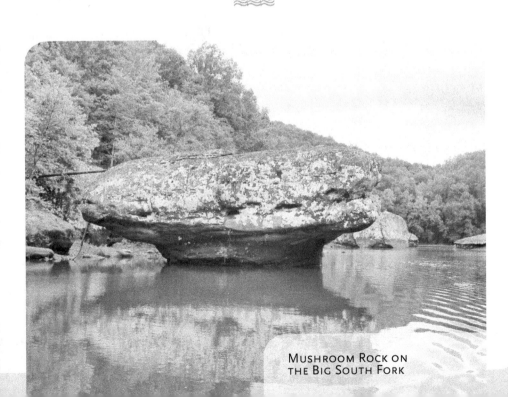

MUSHROOM ROCK ON THE BIG SOUTH FORK

43 BIG SOUTH FORK OF THE CUMBERLAND RIVER (KENTUCKY)

◇ **OVERVIEW** Flowing out of Scott County (TN), the Big South Fork of the Cumberland River flows north through McCreary County (KY) before emptying into Lake Cumberland. One of the most beautiful canoe camping runs in the southeastern United States, the Big South Fork winds through the wooded bluffs and ridges of the Big South Fork National River and Recreation Area (BSFNRRA). An exceptionally scenic river flowing swiftly below stately exposed rock pinnacles, the Big South Fork is dotted with huge boulders midstream and along the banks and padded along either side by steep hillsides of hardwoods and evergreens. Wildflowers brighten the vista in the spring, and wildlife is plentiful.

◇ **MAPS** ONEIDA SOUTH, ONEIDA NORTH, BARTHELL, NEVELSVILLE, BURNSVILLE (USGS); BIG SOUTH FORK NATIONAL RIVER AND RECREATION AREA MAP

Leatherwood Ford to KY 927

Class	II (IV)
Gauge	Web
Level	Min. 200–Max. 1,300/ 3,000 open/decked (cfs)
Gradient	10'
Scenery	A

◇ **DESCRIPTION** Not only will the beauty capture your attention, but the paddling is interesting with as many as five legitimate (and six borderline) Class II rapids (some of them quite long) consisting primarily of nontechnical small ledges and standing waves. The main channel is easily discerned in these rapids, and scouting is normally not required. At moderate to low water, all the Class II rapids can be run with a loaded boat. At higher water, loaded open boats can avail themselves of sneak routes to avoid swamping. The rapids are broken by occasional long, slow stretches. Paddlers can enjoy a day trip on this section, going from Leatherwood Ford (A), to Station Camp (B).

Two Class III–IV rapids are encountered on this section of the Big South Fork. Both are technical, complex, high-velocity chutes that are dangerous at certain water levels. The first is Angel Falls, 1.5 miles into the run, where the river takes an 8-foot drop in closely spaced 1- and 2-foot increments, with the main flow being forced between two large rocks toward the right of the river. After the first two ledges (normally run from the left), converging smaller chutes of water join the main flow from the right, further aerating the water and causing the current to impact a large boulder to the left. A smaller boulder at the bottom of the rapid, in conjunction with the converging currents from the right, causes the current to turn left at the end of the rapid before pooling out. This rapid must be scouted, and different strategies are appropriate at different water levels (though as a point of departure, Angel Falls is usually run far left to left center to right center). Regardless of water level, boats should be emptied of all gear before attempting the run. Portage is possible via a trail on the right 50 yards upstream of the rapid and is strongly recommended at all water levels except for competent, very experienced boaters.

Big South Fork of the Cumberland River (Kentucky)

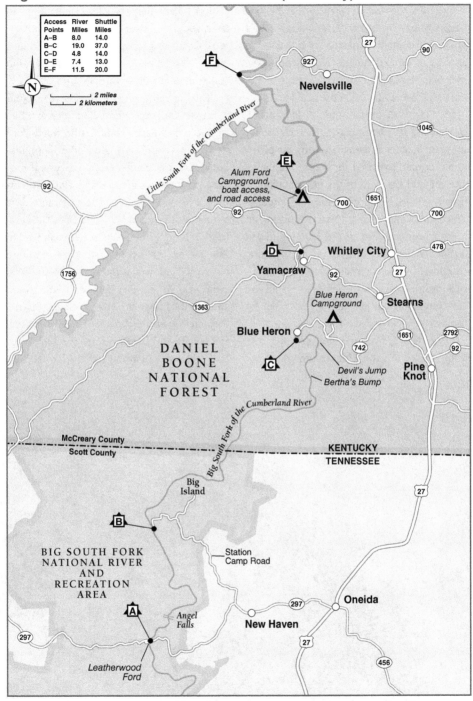

Access Points	River Miles	Shuttle Miles
A–B	8.0	14.0
B–C	19.0	37.0
C–D	4.8	14.0
D–E	7.4	13.0
E–F	11.5	20.0

2 miles
2 kilometers

27
90
927
Nevelsville
1045

Little South Fork of the Cumberland River

92

E
Alum Ford
Campground,
boat access,
and road access
700
1651
700
92
92

D
Whitley City
Yamacraw
1756
92
27
478

1363
Blue Heron
Campground
Stearns

Blue Heron
1651
2792

DANIEL
BOONE
NATIONAL
FOREST
C
742
92

Devil's Jump
Bertha's Bump
**Pine
Knot**

Big South Fork of the Cumberland River

McCreary County
Scott County
KENTUCKY
TENNESSEE

27

Big
Island

B

BIG SOUTH FORK
NATIONAL RIVER
AND
RECREATION
AREA

Station
Camp Road

A
Angel
Falls
297
New Haven
297
Oneida
27
456

Leatherwood
Ford

The Devil's Jump, a Class IV rapid, is closer to the end of the run, just upstream of the Blue Heron Mine. Here the current flows into a house-size boulder from whence it is diverted at an angle through a high-velocity chute. The trick is to align your boat for the chute by riding the pillow off the left of the boulder. This is done at low to moderate water levels by practically setting your bow on a collision course for the giant boulder and then allowing the pillow to divert your bow into the top of the chute. The route to the right of the giant boulder is usually avoided because of a mean hydraulic at the bottom. Once again, all boats should be run without gear and after careful scouting (if you do not understand the dynamics of converging currents, leave this rapid alone). Portage is possible upstream and to the left of the rapid and is recommended at all water levels except for competent, experienced boaters.

The Blue Heron take-out not only has a fine ramp, but the Blue Heron mine and community site has been interpreted by the National Park Service. Allow some time to learn about this river's past while down here. It is fascinating. Yamacraw Landing comes next, and after that, Alum Fork has a ramp and a small, primitive campground.

The Big South Fork is runnable year-round in this section, except for fall in dry years. Day trips can be made from Leatherwood Ford to Station Camp and using other combinations of access points. However, several nice camping locations are available along the run (which can be lengthened to 3 or more days by continuing on down into Lake Cumberland). It is 27 miles from Leatherwood Ford to Blue Heron, 4.8 more to Yamacraw, 7.4 more to Alum Ford, and another 11.5 to the boat ramp near Nevelsville. Between Leatherwood and Devil's Jump, the river averages 80–110 feet but sometimes broadens to as much as 150 feet Below Devil's Jump; the Big South Fork widens to an average of 115–150 feet and

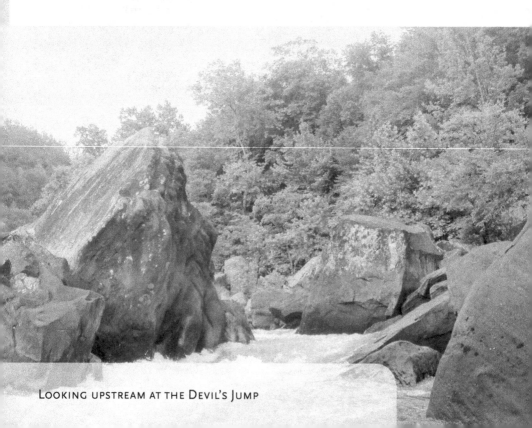

LOOKING UPSTREAM AT THE DEVIL'S JUMP

settles down conspicuously with fewer rapids in evidence. Downstream from Yamacraw, the current comes to a halt as it reaches the lake pool. Dangers to navigation are as described, plus a damaged concrete ford between Blue Heron and Yamacraw that must be portaged on the right, and the potential of the river to rise at an alarming rate after heavy rains (remember this when you set up camp). Because of the remoteness of the Big South Fork, access points are few and far between and connected by narrow roads.

◇ **SHUTTLE** To reach the take-out from Whitley City, take US 27 North 8.8 miles. Turn left onto KY 927 and go 9 miles to dead-end at the boat ramp on the Big South Fork. To reach the put-in from the take-out, return to Whitley City and take US 27 South 17 miles to Oneida,

Tennessee. From Oneida, take TN 297 West 11 miles to Leatherwood Fork access on the right before the bridge over the Big South Fork.

◇ **GAUGE** The USGS gauge is South Fork Cumberland River at Leatherwood Ford, TN. The minimum level is 200 cfs; anything below that and you will be scraping in places. The maximum level is 3,000 cfs.

GPS Coordinates

ACCESS	LATITUDE	LONGITUDE
A	N36° 28.637'	W84° 40.098'
B	N36° 32.934'	W84° 39.900'
C	N36° 40.102'	W84° 32.868'
D	N36° 43.524'	W84° 32.655'
E	N36° 45.826'	W84° 32.807'
F	N36° 50.280'	W84° 35.670'

44 LITTLE SOUTH FORK OF THE CUMBERLAND RIVER

◇ **OVERVIEW** The Little South Fork of the Cumberland River is a Kentucky Wild River. Little used by paddlers due to its seasonal nature and its remoteness, it is nevertheless one of the most beautiful of Kentucky's rivers. Above all, the Little South Fork is amazingly pristine and rugged. Draining the eastern portion of Wayne County and the western portion of McCreary County before emptying into the Big South Fork of the Cumberland River, the Little South Fork runs cool and clear over a rock and mud bottom through steep, wooded hills.

◇ **MAPS** BELL FARM, COOPERSVILLE, NEVELSVILLE (USGS)

Parmleysville to Big South Fork

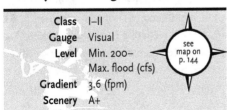

Class	I–II
Gauge	Visual
Level	Min. 200–
	Max. flood (cfs)
Gradient	3.6 (fpm)
Scenery	A+

see map on p. 144

◇ **DESCRIPTION** This truly beautiful watercourse is runnable from November through mid-May downstream from Parmleysville. The stream is primarily Class I with some small shoals and rapids that approach Class II. The river is 30 feet wide in the upstream sections

Little South Fork of the Cumberland River

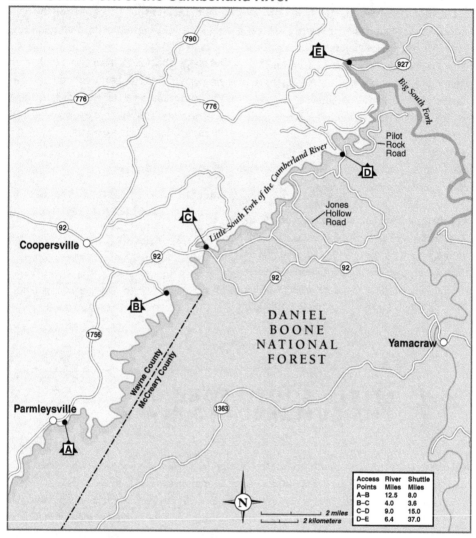

and does not broaden beyond 60 feet as it flows toward its mouth. Access is difficult from all but one or two bridges, and shuttles are long, particularly for the shuttle between the lower river and KY 927, on the Big South Fork. However, the Parmleysville put-in is easy at a low-water bridge. It is a 16.5-mile run between Parmleysville (A) and the KY 92 bridge (C)

(access for KY 92 is on west side of bridge). Exposed rock and a variety of hardwoods grace the usually steep riverbank along with the common proliferation of willows upstream of KY 92. Downstream of KY 92, near Freedom Chapel, the stream enters a massive and beautiful vertical rock-wall gorge. Dangers to navigation include deadfalls and flash flood potential.

✧ **SHUTTLE** From US 27 in Whitley City, take US 27 North to KY 927. Turn left on KY 927 and follow it 9 miles to dead-end at a boat ramp on the Big South Fork near Nevelsville. To reach the uppermost access, take KY 92 West from Whitley City to KY 1756, passing over the Little South Fork on a bridge en route. Turn left on KY 1756 and follow it to veer right on Parmleysville Road. After climbing and descending a big hill, look left for gravel Lonesome Road leading left to a low-water bridge over the Little South Fork.

✧ **GAUGE** Check the Little South Fork when the nearby Big South Fork is running high and muddy.

GPS COORDINATES

ACCESS	LATITUDE	LONGITUDE
A	N36° 40.920'	W84° 44.986'
B	N36° 47.916'	W84° 35.835'
C	N36° 45.503'	W84° 40.350'
D	N36° 47.925'	W84° 35.838'
E	N36° 50.280'	W84° 35.670'

ROCK CREEK

✧ **OVERVIEW** Rock Creek is a small, beautiful creek that drains the southwestern corner of McCreary County near the Tennessee border. The upper section of the creek, above White Oak junction, is protected as a Kentucky Wild River. Unfortunately for paddlers, however, the only paddleable section is from below White Oak junction. Rock Creek runs through the steep, wooded hillsides of the Daniel Boone National Forest. Banks on the roadside of the stream vary in steepness, and the far bank often approaches being vertical. The streamside is dense with scrub vegetation and some trees, with deadfalls not unusual in the upper sections.

✧ **MAPS** BARTHELL SW, BELL FARM, BARTHELL (USGS); BIG SOUTH FORK NATIONAL RIVER AND RECREATION AREA MAP; DANIEL BOONE NATIONAL FOREST MAP, SOUTH SECTION

White Oak Junction to Big South Fork

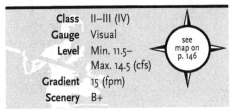

Class	II–III (IV)
Gauge	Visual
Level	Min. 11.5–Max. 14.5 (cfs)
Gradient	15 (fpm)
Scenery	B+

see map on p. 146

✧ **DESCRIPTION** Runnable in the spring and following heavy rain, Rock Creek is a Class II–III, whitewater run with numerous small ledges and a variety of boulders and rocks.

Access is easy with White Oak Road, KY 1363 running along the stream. The logical put-in is at the bridge at Devil's Creek Road with a take-out on the Big South Fork of the Cumberland near Yamacraw. Above Devil's Creek Road, Rock Creek is runnable in spots but would require excessive flow for an unobstructed run. At one spot a half mile upstream of Devil's Creek, the entire stream pools and drops over a ledge to the left under an undercut rock that makes portaging necessary at any water level. For the most part the stream is strewn with boulders and approximately 25–40 feet in width.

Rock Creek

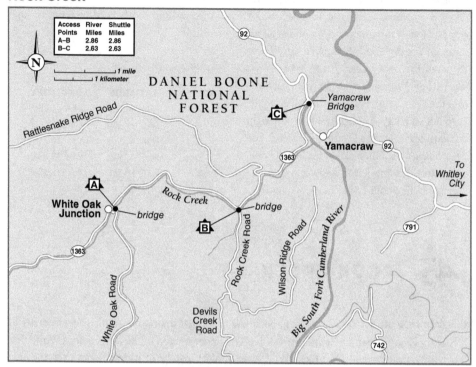

Access Points	River Miles	Shuttle Miles
A–B	2.86	2.86
B–C	2.63	2.63

N

1 mile
1 kilometer

DANIEL BOONE
NATIONAL
FOREST

Rattlesnake Ridge Road

92

C Yamacraw
Bridge

Yamacraw 92

1363

To
Whitley
City

A

White Oak
Junction — bridge

Rock Creek

bridge

B

Rock Creek Road

Wilson Ridge Road

Big South Fork Cumberland River

791

1363

White Oak Road

Devils
Creek
Road

742

✧ **SHUTTLE** To reach the take-out from Whitley City, take US 27 South 1 mile to KY 92. Turn right onto KY 92 West and follow it 6.5 miles to the bridge over the Big South Fork and the Yamacraw boat ramp, accessed just after crossing the bridge.

✧ **GAUGE** The entire run can be scouted from KY 1363. If the Big South Fork is running well above normal flows following heavy rains, consider Rock Creek. Paddlers have used the South Fork Cumberland River at Leatherwood Ford, TN, as a rough gauge. If this gauge is between 11.5 feet and 14.5 feet, then Rock Creek may well be runnable.

GPS Coordinates

ACCESS	LATITUDE	LONGITUDE
A	N36° 42.192'	W84° 35.756'
B	N36° 42.170'	W84° 33.769'
C	N36° 43.529'	W84° 32.679'

46 CUMBERLAND RIVER FROM WOLF CREEK DAM TO THE TENNESSEE BORDER

✧ **OVERVIEW** After passing through the Wolf Creek Dam in Russell County, the Cumberland River turns south through Cumberland and Monroe Counties before crossing once more into Tennessee. This tailwater was created in 1952 with the completion of Wolf Creek Dam. Interestingly, the water discharging from the dam averages 52°F. Compared with other Kentucky rivers of similar size, it is remarkably free of powerboat traffic.

✧ **MAPS** WOLF CREEK DAM, BURKESVILLE, WATERVIEW, BLACKS FERRY, VERNON, CELINA (USGS)

Wolf Creek Dam to Tennessee

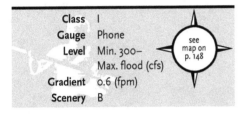

Class	I
Gauge	Phone
Level	Min. 300– Max. flood (cfs)
Gradient	0.6 (fpm)
Scenery	B

see map on p. 148

✧ **DESCRIPTION** Coming cool and clear out of Wolf Creek Dam, the Cumberland is runnable all year here. Flow from the dam dictates river speed. Averaging 200–400 feet in width, access is easy and there are few dangers. Trips of varied lengths are easily made with numerous access points, including a riverside launch on Lower River Road in Burkesville. Although this section of the Cumberland lacks the wilderness quality of the Big South Fork, it nevertheless flows through beautiful, steep woodland and farm country. Mud banks rise on the average 6–12 feet to a floodplain that varies in width and is lined with tall grass and willows. Wind and a few boats are the only hazards to navigation.

✧ **SHUTTLE** To reach the take-out from Burkesville, take KY 90 West 6.2 miles. Turn left onto KY 100 West and follow it 16 miles. Turn left onto KY 214 and go 1.8 miles to reach the ramp on the river. To reach the put-in from the take-out, return to Burkesville and take KY 90 East 10.4 miles. Turn left on KY 1590 and go 2 miles. Turn left onto US 127 North and travel 11 miles, crossing Wolf Creek Dam. Immediately after the dam, turn left onto Dam Road to reach the tailwater ramp next to Kendall Campground.

✧ **GAUGE** The Cumberland is runnable all year. However, the flow rates can vary with the dam release schedule. For the release schedule, call the Wolf Creek Dam Hotline at 800-238-2264, then dial 4, and then 34.

GPS COORDINATES

ACCESS	LATITUDE	LONGITUDE
A	N36° 52.248'	W85° 8.817'
B	N36° 52.280'	W85° 14.640'
C	N36° 51.670'	W85° 19.010'
D	N36° 49.777'	W85° 22.139'
E	N36° 47.172'	W85° 21.928'
F	N36° 44.826'	W85° 22.348'
G	N36° 45.744'	W85° 29.388'
H	N36° 41.160'	W85° 34.010'

Cumberland River: Wolf Creek Dam to the Tennessee Border

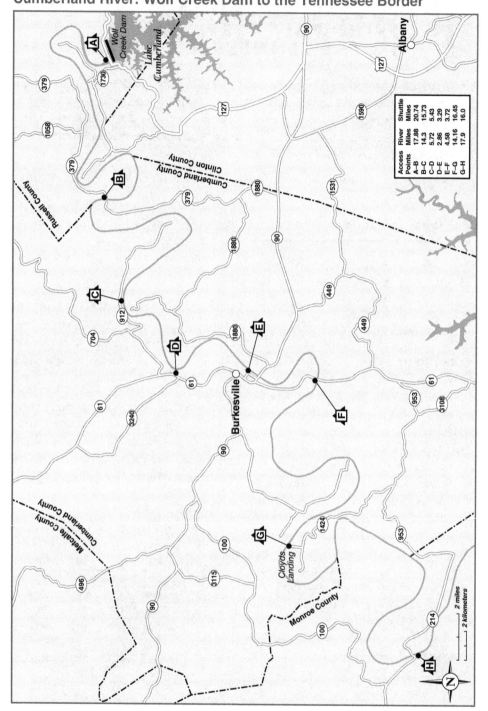

THE SALT RIVER SYSTEM OF THE WESTERN BLUEGRASS

47 SALT RIVER

◆ **OVERVIEW** Originating in Boyle County near Danville, the Salt River flows north and then west, draining the Bluegrass counties of Mercer, Anderson, Spencer, and Bullitt before disappearing into the Fort Knox Military Reservation en route to emptying into the Ohio River near West Point. Runnable downstream of KY 1160 to Taylorsville Lake from late fall to late spring and downstream of Taylorsville Lake almost all year, the Salt is a winding, sycamore-lined stream often bordered by medium-size hills and ridges on one bank and broad fields or grazing land on the other. Current is usually swift, particularly in the winter and spring; access is generally good. However, bona fide ramps and launches are few, save for Taylorsville Lake downstream. Be considerate of landowners near bridges and consider asking for permission to launch. The Salt cannot be paddled into the Fort Knox Military Reservation; therefore, all runs must end at Shepherdsville.

◆ **MAPS** CORNISHVILLE, MCBRAYER, LAWRENCEBURG, GLENSBORO, ASHBROOK, CHAPLIN, BLOOMFIELD, TAYLORSVILLE, WATERFORD, MT. WASHINGTON, BROOKS, SHEPHERDSVILLE (USGS)

A
KY 1160 Bridge to Glensboro

Class	I+
Gauge	Web
Level	Min. 200–Max. flood (cfs)
Gradient	2'
Scenery	B–

47A DESCRIPTION Running over a bottom of sandy mud, the Salt is dotted with dozens of small islands. Banks in the upper sections incline gently but below Taylorsville become increasingly steep and muddy. The level of difficulty is Class I+ in most sections with some tight maneuvering occasionally required to navigate around the islands. Deadfalls and

Salt River: KY 1160 Bridge to Glensboro

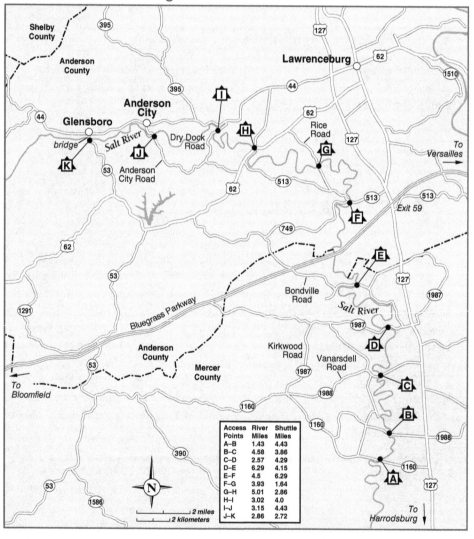

Access Points	River Miles	Shuttle Miles
A–B	1.43	4.43
B–C	4.58	3.86
C–D	2.57	4.29
D–E	6.29	4.15
E–F	4.5	6.29
F–G	3.93	1.64
G–H	5.01	2.86
H–I	3.02	4.0
I–J	3.15	4.43
J–K	2.86	2.72

logjams are numerous and constitute the primary hazards to paddlers. (There is also a 5-foot dam at McBrayer that must be portaged.) Frequent small rapids, ledges, and waves liven up the paddling but should pose no problems. It is 19 miles from the KY 1160 bridge to McBrayer, and 18 miles from McBrayer to Glensboro.

✧ SHUTTLE To reach the take-out from Lawrenceburg, take KY 44 West for 9 miles. Turn left onto KY 53 and follow it south 0.2 mile to the bridge over the Salt River. To reach the put-in from the take-out, backtrack to Lawrenceburg and take US 127 south for 13.3 miles. Turn right onto KY 1160 and follow it west 1.6 miles to the bridge over the Salt River.

✧ GAUGE The USGS gauge is Salt River at Glensboro, KY. Minimum reading should be 200 cfs.

GPS Coordinates

ACCESS	LATITUDE	LONGITUDE
A	N37° 51.175'	W84° 52.884'
B	N37° 51.917'	W84° 52.558'
C	N37° 53.568'	W84° 52.905'
D	N37° 54.924'	W84° 52.623'
E	N37° 56.092'	W84° 53.761'
F	N37° 58.395'	W84° 54.023'
G	N37° 59.428'	W84° 55.170'
H	N37° 59.897'	W84° 57.562'
I	N38° 0.404'	W84° 58.905'
J	N38° 0.221'	W85° 1.225'
K	N38° 0.113'	W85° 3.604'

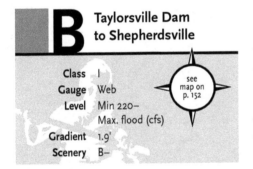

B Taylorsville Dam to Shepherdsville

Class	I
Gauge	Web
Level	Min 220– Max. flood (cfs)
Gradient	1.9'
Scenery	B–

see map on p. 152

47B DESCRIPTION The Salt averages 55–75 feet wide below Taylorsville. There is an Army Corps of Engineers ramp below the Taylorsville Dam. It is 3.5 miles from the dam to Taylorsville, 22 miles from Taylorsville to US 31E, and 15 miles from US 31E to Shepherdsville. Paddlers must take out before reaching Fort Knox. In Shepherdsville, paddlers can access the river via the park on First Street, just south of the KY 61 bridge over the Salt.

✧ SHUTTLE The take-out is located at the park on First Street, just south of the KY 61 bridge over the Salt River. To reach the put-in from the take-out, take KY 44 East for 23 miles through Taylorsville. Turn right onto KY 2239 and follow it 1.5 miles. Turn right onto Tailwater Road to dead-end at an access below Taylorsville Lake Dam.

✧ GAUGE The USGS gauge is Salt River at Shepherdsville. The minimum reading should be 220 cfs.

GPS Coordinates

ACCESS	LATITUDE	LONGITUDE
M	N38° 0.793'	W85° 18.474'
N	N38° 1.678'	W85° 20.510'
O	N38° 1.370'	W85° 25.860'
P	N38° 0.762'	W85° 30.776'
Q	N37° 59.691'	W85° 33.522'
R	N37° 59.173'	W85° 43.262'

Salt River: Taylorsville Dam to Shepherdsville

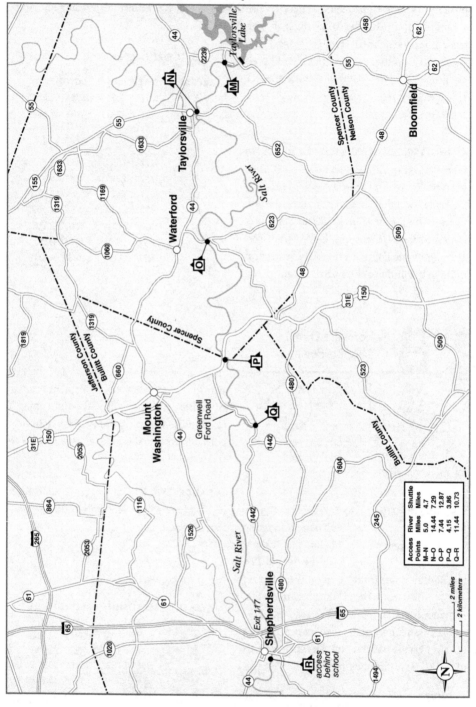

48 PLUM CREEK

✧ **OVERVIEW** Plum Creek originates in southwestern Shelby County and flows south through Spencer County before emptying into the Salt River west of Taylorsville. Only runnable after heavy rains, the Plum rollercoasters over a seemingly continuous series of ledges ranging from several inches to 3 feet in height.

✧ **MAPS** FISHERVILLE, WATERFORD (USGS)

Wilsonville to Waterford

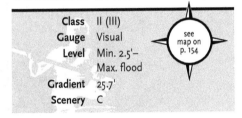

Class	II (III)
Gauge	Visual
Level	Min. 2.5'–
	Max. flood
Gradient	25.7'
Scenery	C

see map on p. 154

✧ **DESCRIPTION** Flowing over a rock bed between high, well-defined banks of varying steepness, Plum Creek is unique among high-water streams (that is, streams that can only be run after exceptionally heavy rains). First, there are practically no deadfalls, and the channel is almost uniformly unobstructed. Second, the geology of the riverbed limits lateral erosion and keeps the stream neatly within the confines of its banks, even at very high levels.

Plum Creek can be run from Hochstrasser Road at the Shelby–Spencer County line all the way to its mouth at the Salt River. Above KY 155, however, numerous fences spanning the stream make paddling both dangerous and bothersome. Below KY 155 about a third of a mile is a low-water bridge. Beyond this point, the river is normally clear of strainers (man-made or otherwise).

The run is a good, solid Class II with an average gradient of 25 feet per mile and would

have to be upgraded to Class III at higher water levels (above 3 feet on the gauge on the upstream side of the KY 3192 bridge). The whitewater is challenging but not particularly technical, consisting of nearly continuous waves, small holes, and lots of vertical drops. At higher levels, eddies are few and far between. There are several major rapids between the KY 1319 bridge and the KY 44 bridge that can be easily scouted from KY 1060, which runs parallel to the stream. The principal attraction of Plum Creek is its whitewater and proximity to Louisville (35 miles). Scenery along the creek is only passable at best, with habitation all along its banks and less-than-average vegetation. Surrounding countryside consists of rolling terrain spotted with small farms. Dangers to navigation include several low-water fords and small dams. Because the nature (and difficulty) of the run varies markedly at different water levels, thorough scouting is advised.

Be very judicious when parking off KY 1319, whether it is off Kings Church Road ford or the KY 1319 bridge. Ask for landowner permission. The lowermost take-out is at Spencer County's Waterford Park, just upstream of the KY 44 bridge.

✧ **SHUTTLE** To reach the take-out from Taylorsville, take KY 44 West 5.4 miles to the park on the right just before the bridge over Plum Creek. To reach the put-in from the take-out, keep west on KY 44, bridging Plum Creek, then turn right onto KY 1060 and follow it for 5.2 miles. Keep straight, joining KY 1319, and follow it 2.8 miles to KY 3192. Turn left onto KY 3192 and follow it 0.9 mile to the bridge over Plum Creek. Be very careful parking here and consider entering the creek at the KY 155 bridge, just upstream of the KY 3192 bridge.

◆ GAUGE The gauge is on the KY 3192 bridge at upper Plum Creek. The gauge should be at least 2.5 feet.

GPS Coordinates

ACCESS	LATITUDE	LONGITUDE
A	N38° 7.513'	W85° 24.355'
B	N38° 6.418'	W85° 26.294'
C	N38° 2.344'	W85° 26.199'

Plum Creek

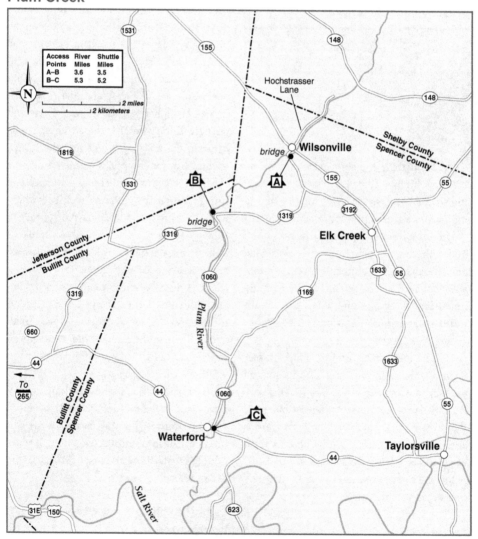

Access Points	River Miles	Shuttle Miles
A–B	3.6	3.5
B–C	5.3	5.2

49 FLOYDS FORK OF THE SALT RIVER

✧ **OVERVIEW** A main tributary of the Salt River and a state Bluewater Trail, Floyds Fork flows southwest along the Oldham–Shelby County line, across western Jefferson County, and into Bullitt County, where it joins the Salt River near Shepherdsville. Access is good, especially in Jefferson and Shelby Counties, where the banks are not particularly steep. Luckily for today's paddlers, the Parklands of Floyds Fork was created. It is a series of five parks encompassing roughly 4,000 acres along the river's banks. A series of accesses placed along the stream at intervals in the Parklands of Floyds Fork has turned Floyds Fork into a true easy-to-reach paddling access for greater Louisville. This park also features trails linking the paddling accesses, making bike shuttles viable and even fun.

✧ **MAPS** Crestwood, Fisherville, Jeffersontown, Mt. Washington (USGS)

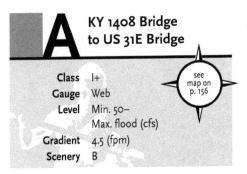

A KY 1408 Bridge to US 31E Bridge

Class	I+
Gauge	Web
Level	Min. 50–
	Max. flood (cfs)
Gradient	4.5 (fpm)
Scenery	B

see map on p. 156

49A **DESCRIPTION** Runnable downstream of KY 1408 from mid-fall through the spring, Floyds Fork rolls alternately beneath steep hills and ridges. What once were fields and pastureland have been replaced in many places by Louisville's exurbs. Current is swift, and the stream is punctuated with small ledges, shoals, and many brush islands. The river averages 35–55 feet in width. The stream's level of difficulty is Class I+, with good paddling techniques necessary to navigate around many of the islands. Dangers to navigation include numerous deadfalls and logjams.

✧ **SHUTTLE** To reach the take-out from Exit 17 on I-265, southeast of Louisville, take

US 150/Bardstown Road south for 4.4 miles. Turn left into Broad Run Park and the Broad Run Valley paddling access. To reach the put-in, return to Exit 17 and take I-265 East 12 miles to Exit 29. Follow Henry Road east 0.3 mile, then turn right on Aiken Road and follow it 6.3 miles. Turn left onto KY 1408 and follow it for 0.9 mile to the bridge over Floyds Fork.

✧ **GAUGE** The USGS gauge is Floyds Fork at Fisherville, KY. Minimum reading should be 200 cfs.

GPS Coordinates

ACCESS	LATITUDE	LONGITUDE
A	N38° 18.446'	W85° 27.008'
B	N38° 17.148'	W85° 28.088'
C	N38° 15.931'	W85° 27.824'
D	N38° 13.810'	W85° 28.060'
E	N38° 12.957'	W85° 28.628'
F	N38° 11.253'	W85° 28.549'
G	N38° 9.104'	W85° 30.131'
H	N38° 7.942'	W85° 31.082'
I	N38° 6.230'	W85° 32.710'
J	N38° 5.160'	W85° 33.310'

Floyds Fork of the Salt River: KY 1408 Bridge to US 31E Bridge

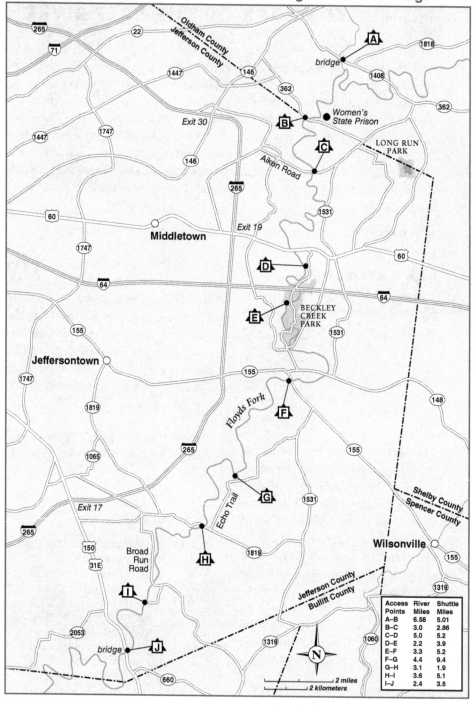

Access Points	River Miles	Shuttle Miles
A–B	6.58	5.01
B–C	3.0	2.86
C–D	5.0	5.2
D–E	2.2	3.9
E–F	3.3	5.2
F–G	4.4	9.4
G–H	3.1	1.9
H–I	3.6	5.1
I–J	2.4	3.5

B US 31E Bridge to Salt River in Shepherdsville

Class	I+
Gauge	Web
Level	Min. 50–Max. flood (cfs)
Gradient	3.9'
Scenery	B–

49B **DESCRIPTION** The river broadens, averaging 45–65 feet wide. It is 12 miles from the US 31E bridge to the KY 1526 bridge and 11.5 miles farther to the access point in Shepherdsville, which is on the main Salt River.

◇ **GAUGE** The USGS gauge is Floyds Fork at Fisherville, KY. Minimum reading should be 50 cfs.

GPS COORDINATES

ACCESS	LATITUDE	LONGITUDE
I	N38° 5.160'	W85° 33.310'
J	N38° 2.096'	W85° 39.491'
K	N38° 0.250'	W85° 40.940'
L	N37° 59.173'	W85° 43.262'

Floyds Fork of the Salt River: US 31E Bridge to Salt River in Shepherdsville

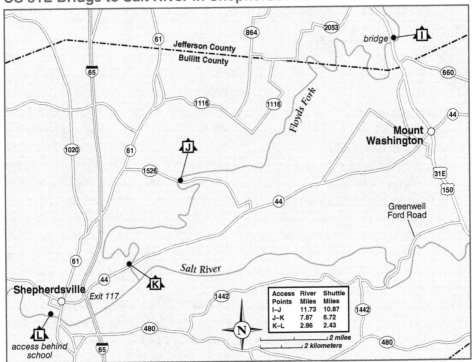

50 ROLLING FORK OF THE SALT RIVER

◇ **OVERVIEW** Flowing northwest out of Casey County, the Rolling Fork of the Salt River drains portions of Marion, Larue, Nelson, Bullitt, and Hardin Counties before joining the Salt River deep inside the Fort Knox Military Reservation. Running over a mud and rock bottom and between wall-like mud banks carved by lateral erosion, the Rolling Fork is runnable downstream of the US 68 bridge from November to May. Be warned that floating the Rolling Fork through Fort Knox is strictly prohibited.

◇ **MAPS** LEBANON WEST, RAYWICK, HOWARDSTOWN, NEW HAVEN, NELSONVILLE, LEBANON JUNCTION (USGS)

KY 68 Bridge near Lebanon to Lebanon Junction

Class	I+
Gauge	Web
Level	Min. 140– Max. flood (cfs)
Gradient	2.2'
Scenery	B–C

◇ **DESCRIPTION** Largely, the Rolling Fork meanders beside broad fields on one side of the stream and rolling hills (usually grazing land) on the other. Above the mud walls that contain the river, the banks are brushy and tree lined. Grass and brush islands are common in the stream. The most scenic section of the Rolling Fork is between the Marion County line and New Haven, where there is a boat ramp off US 52, and where the river temporarily departs the farm plains and winds beneath the tall, rugged knobs (a "knob" is larger than a big hill and smaller than a mountain and is so named because of characteristically steep sides and rounded top) of southern Nelson and northern Larue Counties. In this area, the precipitous hillsides are densely forested, and some exposed rock is visible both in the river gorge and high on the ridges. Emerging from the knobs near New Haven, the Rolling Fork continues through hilly farmland until it disappears among the wooded, rolling hills of Fort Knox. The abundance of farmland can stain the Rolling Fork after prolonged rains. Its level of difficulty is Class I+ between US 68 and the Lebanon Junction. Access points are numerous, allowing runs of varying lengths. Navigational dangers are limited to deadfalls, logjams, and several brush islands that necessitate good boat control. The Rolling Fork enters Fort Knox Military Reservation shortly beyond Lebanon Junction. Paddling through the reservation is prohibited. It is 18 miles from the US 68 bridge to Raywick, 17 miles from Raywick to the KY 84 bridge, 18 miles from the KY 84 bridge to New Haven, and 29 miles from New Haven to Lebanon Junction.

◇ **SHUTTLE** To reach the take-out from New Haven, take KY 52 West 11 miles. Turn right onto US 62 East and go 1 mile. Turn left onto KY 61 North and follow it 4.7 miles, passing I-65 to enter Lebanon Junction. Turn left on Main Street and go 0.5 mile. Turn left onto KY 434/Coleburg Road and follow it 1.3 miles

Rolling Fork of the Salt River:
KY 68 Bridge near Lebanon to Lebanon Junction

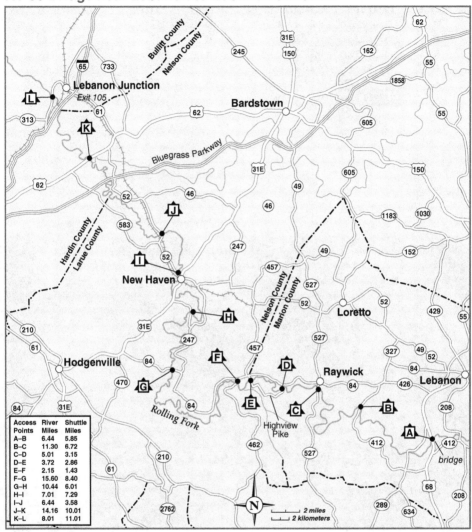

Access Points	River Miles	Shuttle Miles
A–B	6.44	5.85
B–C	11.30	6.72
C–D	5.01	3.15
D–E	3.72	2.86
E–F	2.15	1.43
F–G	15.60	8.40
G–H	10.44	6.01
H–I	7.01	7.29
I–J	6.44	3.58
J–K	14.16	10.01
K–L	8.01	11.01

to the bridge over the Rolling Fork. To reach the put-in from the take-out, backtrack to New Haven and take KY 52 East 7.5 miles. Turn right onto KY 527 and follow it 4.8 miles to turn left onto KY 84. Follow KY 84 east 4.1 miles, then keep straight to join KY 427 for 3.7 miles to reach US 68. Turn right and follow US 68 west 3.3 miles to the bridge over the Rolling Fork.

◇ **GAUGE** The USGS gauge is Rolling Fork near Boston. The minimum reading should be 140 cfs.

GPS Coordinates

ACCESS	LATITUDE	LONGITUDE	ACCESS	LATITUDE	LONGITUDE
A	N37° 30.470'	W85° 17.695'	G	N37° 34.350'	W85° 36.270'
B	N37° 32.324'	W85° 22.779'	H	N37° 37.572'	W85° 34.756'
C	N37° 33.300'	W85° 25.850'	I	N37° 39.727'	W85° 35.808'
D	N37° 33.340'	W85° 28.437'	J	N37° 41.893'	W85° 36.970'
E	N37° 33.772'	W85° 30.675'	K	N37° 46.019'	W85° 42.252'
F	N37° 33.734'	W85° 31.594'	L	N37° 49.381'	W85° 44.856'

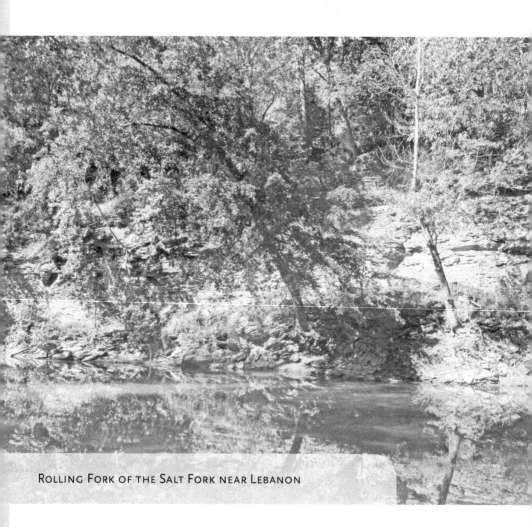

ROLLING FORK OF THE SALT FORK NEAR LEBANON

51 BEECH FORK OF THE ROLLING FORK OF THE SALT RIVER

◇ **OVERVIEW** Beech Fork originates in eastern Marion County, flows northwest into Washington County, where it joins the Chaplin River, and then turns southwest through Nelson County before finally emptying into the Rolling Fork of the Salt River near Boston, Kentucky.

◇ **MAPS** Bardstown, Cravens, Lebanon Junction (USGS)

KY 49 to Boston

Class	I (III+)
Gauge	Web
Level	Min. 150–Max. flood (cfs)
Gradient	1.4'
Scenery	C+

◇ **DESCRIPTION** An extremely winding river, the Beech Fork is runnable from November to early June from KY 49 to its mouth. Tree-lined and having mud banks of varying steepness while flowing over a mud bottom, the Beech Fork (in its runnable section) snakes through the modest knobs of

Beech Fork of the Rolling Fork of the Salt River

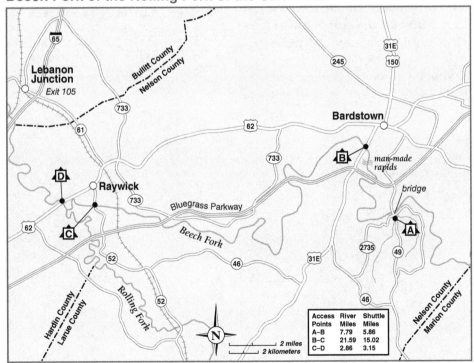

Access Points	River Miles	Shuttle Miles
A–B	7.79	5.86
B–C	21.59	15.02
C–D	2.86	3.15

central Nelson County, past the distilleries on the southern edge of Bardstown, and on to the broad, gently rolling farm plains of Boston. Its level of difficulty is Class I, with the exception of a man-made Class III+ (a collapsed boulder dam) one-quarter of a mile upstream of the US 31E bridge. The overall drop here is about 5 feet. This rapid can be safely run but changes incredibly with varying water levels and should always be scouted. The rapid is dominated by a vault-size boulder right in the middle of the river at the bottom of a 4-foot drop. To its left (as you look downstream) is a mean hole, particularly at higher water levels. When the water is up, there is a nice route on the far left; otherwise, choose your own poison or carry around. This river has been modified by the city of Bardstown around this rapid in order to create a play wave at proper water levels. Other hazards to navigation include numerous brush islands, deadfalls, and some logjams. A good day trip extends 8 miles from KY 49 to Bardstown and the US 31E bridge.

◊ **SHUTTLE** To reach the take-out from Exit 21 on the Blue Grass Parkway, south of Bardstown, take the Blue Grass west for 11 miles to Exit 10 and follow KY 52 west 2 miles to reach US 62. Turn left and take US 62 West 1.4 miles to the bridge over the Beech Fork. To reach the put-in from the take-out, return to Exit 21 and head north on US 31E 1.7 miles. Turn right onto Muir Avenue in Bardstown and go 0.2 mile. Turn right on 4th Avenue and follow it 0.4 mile, where it becomes Gilkey Run Road. Stay on Gilkey Run Road for 0.8 mile, then turn right onto KY 49 South and follow it 2.5 miles to cross the bridge over Beech Fork. Turn left just past the bridge. Turn left again onto Roberts Road, then immediately turn left again onto a dirt access road.

◊ **GAUGE** The USGS gauge is Beech Fork at Bardstown. The minimum reading should be 150 cfs.

GPS Coordinates

ACCESS	LATITUDE	LONGITUDE
A	N37° 45.456'	W85° 27.516'
B	N37° 47.812'	W85° 28.811'
C	N37° 45.923'	W85° 40.768'
D	N37° 46.020'	W85° 42.210'

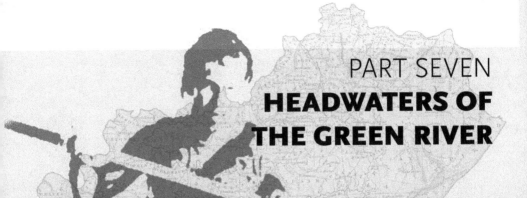

PART SEVEN
HEADWATERS OF THE GREEN RIVER

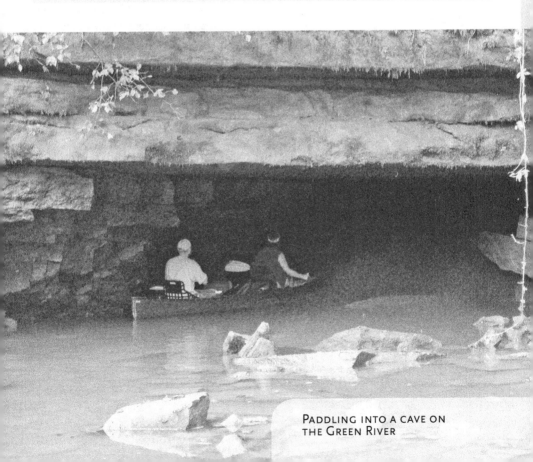

PADDLING INTO A CAVE ON THE GREEN RIVER

52   GREEN RIVER

✧ **OVERVIEW** The Green River is one of Kentucky's largest, longest, and most navigable rivers. Originating in southwestern Lincoln County, the Green River flows west, creating Green River Lake and draining 12 counties before emptying into the Ohio River across from Evansville, Indiana. Although most of the Green River is paddleable all year, certain sections are far more inviting than others. For this reason, the river has been divided into sections. (The lower Green River, from Houchins Ferry at Livermore to the mouth of the Green River at the Rough River, is found in "Part Eight, Streams of the Western Coal Fields.")

✧ **MAPS** LIBERTY, PHIL, DUNNVILLE, KNIFELY, CANE VALLEY, GRESHAM, GREENSBURG, SUMMERSVILLE, HUDGINS, CENTER, CANMER, MUNFORDVILLE, CUB RUN, MAMMOTH CAVE (USGS); MAMMOTH CAVE NATIONAL PARK MAP; GREEN RIVER LAKE ARMY CORPS OF ENGINEERS MAP

A   Liberty to Green River Lake

Class	I+
Gauge	Visual
Level	Min. 120– Max. flood (cfs)
Gradient	3.8'
Scenery	B

52A **DESCRIPTION** This upper section of the Green is not often paddled but is very pleasant. Running through farmland and along some steep, wooded hills, the river is tree lined and flows swiftly. Banks are of mud and vary in steepness. At low water, sandbars and brush islands are common. Although farms line the floodplain, the river itself is fairly secluded, and signs of human habitation are surprisingly few. Some modest but interesting exposed rock formations combine with rippling, playful Class I+ water to keep the paddling interesting. Access is good in most places, and navigational hazards are limited to deadfalls and occasional logjams. This section is runnable from November through mid-June. It is 15 miles from Liberty to KY 1640 and 9 miles from KY 1640 to Neatsville. Private property limits paddler-camping possibilities on the river, but campers will find several options available by continuing on to Green River Lake. The last 19 miles of this run, all below Neatsville, are on Green River Lake.

✧ **SHUTTLE** To reach the take-out from Clementsville, take KY 551 West 13.7 miles. Turn right on Egypt Road and go 1.1 miles. Turn right on Holmes Bend Road and follow it 2.6 miles to Holmes Bend Boat Dock on Green River Lake. To reach the put-in from the take-out, backtrack to Clementsville and take KY 70 East 9.4 miles. Turn left on US 127 and travel 2.6 miles to the park and boat ramp on the east side of Liberty.

✧ **GAUGE** The gauge to check for the upper Green is Green River near McKinney, KY. The minimum reading should be 120 cfs. Green River Lake can be paddled year-round.

Green River: Liberty to Green River Lake

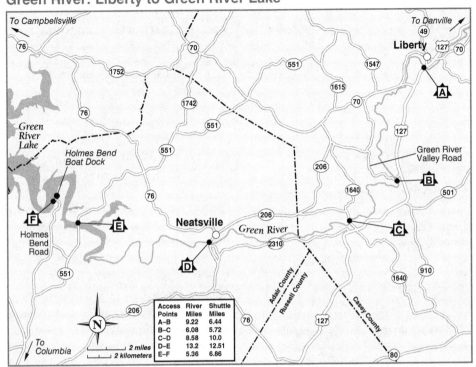

Access Points	River Miles	Shuttle Miles
A–B	9.22	6.44
B–C	6.08	5.72
C–D	8.58	10.0
D–E	13.2	12.51
E–F	5.36	6.86

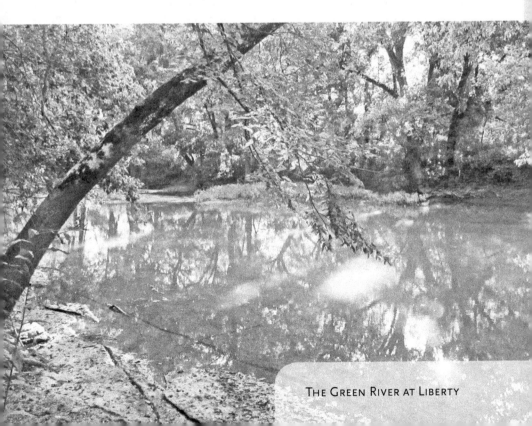

THE GREEN RIVER AT LIBERTY

GPS COORDINATES

ACCESS	LATITUDE	LONGITUDE
A	N37° 18.604'	W84° 56.464'
B	N37° 18.604'	W84° 56.464'
C	N37° 12.375'	W85° 0.458'

ACCESS	LATITUDE	LONGITUDE
D	N37° 11.538'	W85° 7.881'
E	N37° 12.371'	W85° 14.848'
F	N37° 13.355'	W85° 16.129'

B Green River Lake Dam to Munfordville

Class	I+
Gauge	Web, phone
Level	Min. 200– Max. flood (cfs)
Gradient	1'
Scenery	B

52B **DESCRIPTION** This is a popular paddling section, and several trip combinations are available. Flow in this section depends on releases from the Green River Lake Dam (the U.S. Army Corps of Engineers has provided adequate water during warm-weather months for paddling). More exposed rock is visible in this section, surrounding terrain is a bit more rugged, and the river is more secluded than in the previous section. Watch for a tall fall entering river right. Averaging 60 feet in width below the dam, the river widens perceptibly to 100–110 feet by the time it reaches Munfordville. Riffles and small rapids enliven the paddling but do not exceed Class I+. Access is good, including a newer access at Wilson Park, 4 miles upstream of Munfordville. Interestingly, a riverside trail links this park and paddler access to Munfordville, allowing a bike shuttle. Deadfalls and an occasional brush jam are the only navigational hazards at normal water levels. Access points in Roachville, Greensburg, the KY 88 bridge, and the US 31E bridge, as well as Wilson Park, allow for varied trips. Canoe and kayak rentals and shuttle services operate on this stretch of the Green.

⟡ SHUTTLE The take-out is located in downtown Munfordville, at the ramp on River Road, just downstream of the US 31W bridge over the Green River. River Road is accessed from Main Street/US 31W. To reach the put-in from the take-out, take US 31W south 1 mile. Turn left on KY 88 East and stay with it for 24 miles to KY 61. Turn right on KY 61 South and follow it 1.6 miles. Turn left on US 68 East and go 9 miles to Campbellsville. Turn right on KY 55 South and follow it 7.5 miles. Turn left into Tailwater Recreation Area and a boat ramp below Green River Dam.

⟡ GAUGE The USGS gauge is Green River at Munfordville. The minimum reading should be 200 cfs. In addition, the water release information for Green River Lake Dam can be obtained by calling 270-465-8824.

GPS COORDINATES

ACCESS	LATITUDE	LONGITUDE
G	N37° 14.513'	W85° 20.638'
H	N37° 14.120'	W85° 25.469'
I	N37° 14.666'	W85° 28.776'
J	N37° 15.964'	W85° 34.981'
K	N37° 18.064'	W85° 40.291'
L	N37° 18.984'	W85° 46.112'
M	N37° 17.865'	W85° 51.039'
N	N37° 15.971'	W85° 53.342'

Green River: Green River Lake Dam to Munfordville

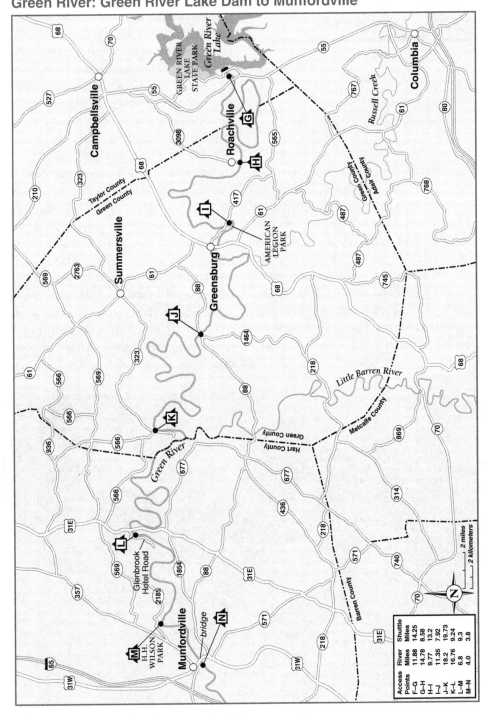

Access Points	River Miles	Shuttle Miles
F–G	11.88	14.25
G–H	14.78	8.58
H–I	9.77	13.2
I–J	11.35	7.92
J–K	18.2	19.73
K–L	16.76	9.24
L–M	6.8	9.3
M–N	4.0	3.8

C Munfordville to Houchins Ferry

Class	I+
Gauge	Web
Level	Min. 200–Max. flood (cfs)
Gradient	1'
Scenery	B

52C **DESCRIPTION** This section of the Green River is also extremely popular, and it runs in large part through Mammoth Cave National Park. Scenery remains essentially the same as for the river section just described, except that beautiful forests supplant the cornfields once the Green River enters the park, and less exposed rock is evident. Wildlife is abundant in this area, with great variety visible to careful observers. Channeled by the steep surrounding hills, the river averages 70–100 feet wide until it reaches Mammoth Ferry, where it broadens to 130 feet as it encounters the backwater pool of the Brownsville Dam. This point also marks the end of any current or riffles for this section. Needless to say, the Green River here runs through cave country, and at least two caves can be scouted at water's edge. A small cave located a half mile downstream of Dennison Ferry on the left bank can actually be paddled into for approximately 40 feet.

Farther downstream, about a mile beyond Mammoth Ferry and 200 feet off the river to the left, is a small cave with a beautiful, clear pool of icy water. Canoe camping is allowed throughout the park, but a backcountry fire and camping permit must be obtained from the park rangers (at no charge). Access to the river is good. Deadfalls are the only navigational hazards. This section is runnable all year when the dam is releasing. Shorter runs can be made from Dennison Ferry and Mammoth Ferry, access points within Mammoth

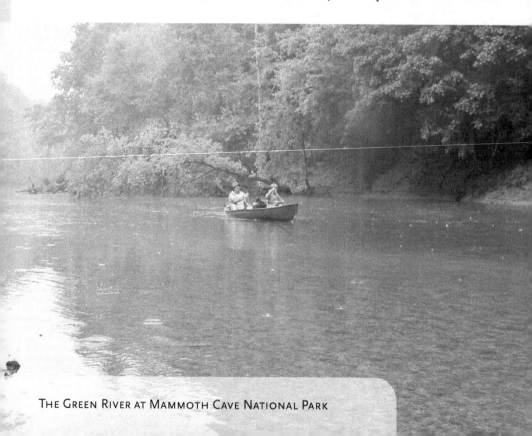

THE GREEN RIVER AT MAMMOTH CAVE NATIONAL PARK

Green River: Munfordville to Houchins Ferry

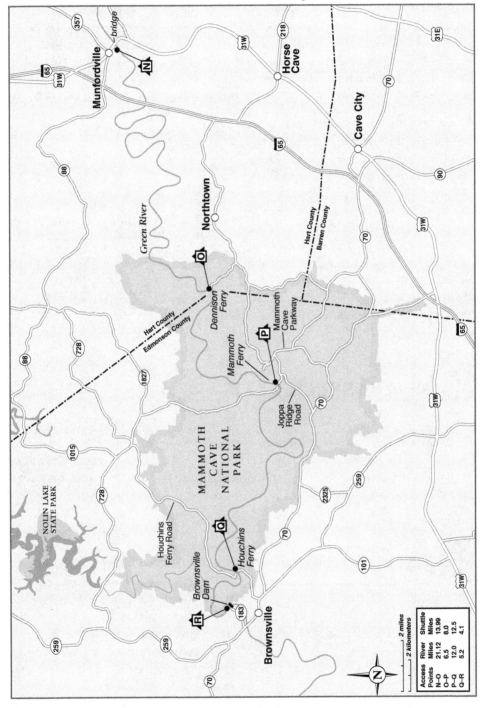

Cave National Park. Outfitters also operate along this stretch of river. It is 21 miles from Munfordville to Dennison Ferry access on the east side of Mammoth Cave National Park and 7 miles from Dennison Ferry to Mammoth Ferry. It is 12 miles from Mammoth Ferry to Houchins Ferry.

SHUTTLE The take-out is located in Brownsville. The boat ramp is located on Old Ferry Road, just downstream of the bridge over the Green River, accessed by heading north on Main Street. To reach the put-in from the take-out, take KY 70 East 12.3 miles, then veer right and join KY 255/Mammoth Cave Parkway and follow it 2.4 miles to I-65. Merge onto I-65 North and go 17 miles to Exit 65. Head south on US 31W 1.5 miles into Munfordville and the ramp on River Road just before crossing the bridge over the Green River.

GAUGE The USGS gauge is Green River at Munfordville; the water release information for Green River Lake Dam can be obtained by calling 270-465-8824. Also, Mammoth Cave National Park operates a water information line: 270-758-2166. They note whether the water level at Green River is above 10 feet, at which level the park discourages the launching of self-propelled watercraft.

GPS COORDINATES

ACCESS	LATITUDE	LONGITUDE
N	N37° 15.971'	W85° 53.342'
O	N37° 12.980'	W86° 2.910'
P	N37° 10.769'	W86° 6.736'
Q	N37° 12.122'	W86° 14.250'
R	N37° 12.299'	W86° 15.621'

53 RUSSELL CREEK

OVERVIEW Overshadowed by a plethora of nearby paddling destinations, Russell Creek offers solitude and good scenery. From its origins in eastern Adair County, Russell Creek flows northwest, gaining enough tributaries to become floatable at Milltown. From here, the Russell meanders north to reach the Green River.

MAPS EXIE, GRESHAM (USGS)

A Milltown to Russell Creek Road

Class	I+
Gauge	Web
Level	Min. 150 –Max. N/A (cfs)
Gradient	5'
Scenery	B

53A DESCRIPTION Russell Creek is generally runnable from late fall to midsummer and following heavy rains. Fishing is reputed to be good. The Class I waters, generally 30–40 feet wide and bordered by both mud and rock banks, offer enough riffles to keep you moving between pools, finally spilling into the Green River southwest of Greensburg.

The uppermost put-in is less commonly used. Occasional limestone bluffs rise from heavily wooded banks with sycamores aplenty. These thick woods obscure rolling farmlands that lie beyond a paddler's view. Watch for

Russell Creek

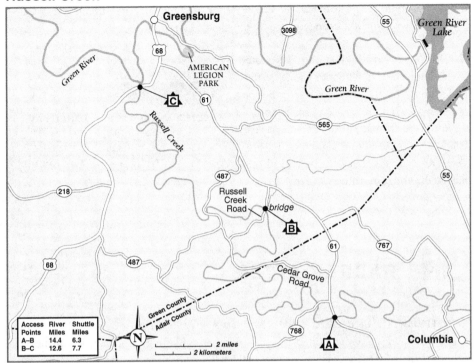

Access Points	River Miles	Shuttle Miles
A–B	14.4	6.3
B–C	12.6	7.7

2 miles

2 kilometers

downed trees around tight bends. This section crosses bridges twice between its beginning and end.

◇ **SHUTTLE** To access the take-out from Greensburg, take US 68 South 1.4 miles to veer left onto KY 61 South for 5.7 miles. Turn right onto Russell Creek Road and follow it 0.8 mile to reach the bridge over Russell Creek. To reach the put-in from the take-out, backtrack to KY 61 and turn right, following KY 61 south 5.5 miles to the bridge over Russell Creek.

◇ **GAUGE** The USGS gauge is Russell Creek near Columbia. The minimum reading should be 175 cfs.

B
Russell Creek Road to KY 68

Class	I+
Gauge	Web
Level	Min. 175 –Max. N/A (cfs)
Gradient	1.2'
Scenery	B

53B DESCRIPTION Russell Creek Road (B) is a more commonly used access. More feeder branches widen the creek a bit and open the canopy in places. Pools are more common than above Russell Creek Road. KY 487 is a seldom-used alternative put-in for a shorter run. The Green River is located just downstream of the

KY 68 take-out. Runs can be extended onto the Green, though the next take-out on the Green is 7 miles down at the KY 88 bridge.

✧ **SHUTTLE** To reach the take-out from Greensburg, take US 68 South 3 miles to the bridge over Russell Creek. To reach the put-in from the take-out, backtrack 1.1 miles on US 68 North, then turn right onto KY 61 East and follow it 5.7 miles to turn right onto Russell Creek Road. Follow Russell Creek Road 0.8 mile to the bridge over Russell Creek.

✧ **GAUGE** The USGS gauge is Russell Creek near Columbia. The minimum reading should be 175 cfs.

GPS COORDINATES

ACCESS	LATITUDE	LONGITUDE
A	N37° 7.168'	W85° 23.613'
B	N37° 10.196'	W85° 26.106'
C	N37° 13.640'	W85° 30.670'

54 BARREN RIVER

✧ **OVERVIEW** The Barren River is one of Kentucky's big rivers. Originating in southern Monroe and Allen Counties near the Tennessee border southeast of Bowling Green, it makes up the main drainage system for a large, four-county area and finally empties into the Green River southeast of Morgantown. It could be very effectively argued that Kentucky's longest and largest river should indeed be the Barren and not the Green. At their confluence, the Barren is easily the larger of the two rivers. Below Barren River Dam, the river can be run all year, with easy access at several points. Deadfalls and occasional sandbars at low water are the only hazards to navigation.

✧ **MAPS** LUCAS, MEADOR, PARKVILLE, BOWLING GREEN SOUTH,
BOWLING GREEN NORTH, HADLEY, RIVERSIDE (USGS)

A Barren River Lake Dam to Bowling Green

Class	I (II)
Gauge	Phone
Level	Min. 170–Max. flood (cfs)
Gradient	1.3'
Scenery	B

54A **DESCRIPTION** Runnable all year round from the dam, the Barren River is especially nice and averages 40–60 feet in width upstream from the mouth of Drakes Creek. Along banks of varying steepness, tree roots are exposed by lateral erosion, and the river is more winding. Islands suitable for canoe camping at medium to low water levels are not uncommon. Vegetation is often lush and many hardwoods are in evidence. Occasionally the banks rise steeply with some exposed rock. Between the mouth of Drakes Creek and Jennings Creek, the Barren River is still wide but a little more scenic and interesting for paddling. Running over sand, rock, and clay banks through a deep bed, the river averages from 90 to 150 feet in width. Watch for a Class II man-made rapid on the loop of the river passing through downtown Bowling Green. However,

Barren River: Barren River Lake Dam to Bowling Green

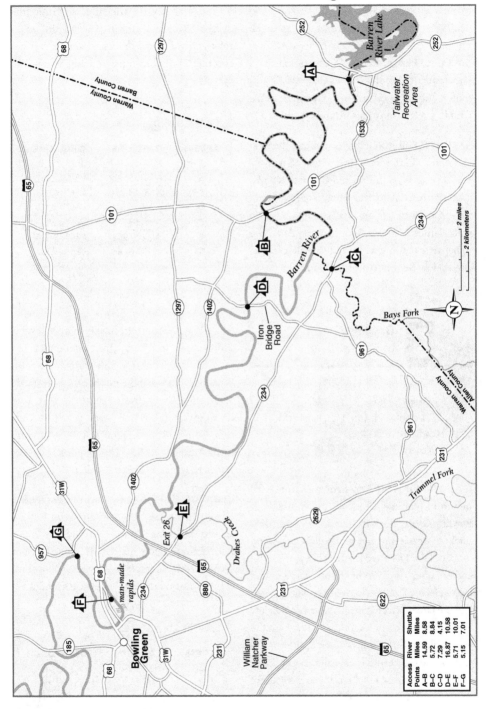

Access Points	River Miles	Shuttle Miles
A–B	14.59	8.58
B–C	5.72	8.84
C–D	7.29	4.15
D–E	16.87	10.58
E–F	5.71	10.01
F–G	5.15	7.01

there is an access just a short ways above the manmade rapid at Weldon Pete Park, off Old Louisville Road. Other accesses are at G. H. Freeman Park, also off Old Louisville Road; the KY 101 bridge, where KY 234 crosses Bays Fork (put-in only); and Drakes Creek on KY 234 (put-in only). A good but long day trip from the dam to the KY 101 bridge extends 15 miles.

✧ **SHUTTLE** To reach the take-out on the west side of Bowling Green (G) from Exit 26 on I-65, take KY 234 West in Bowling Green to KY 185. Turn right on KY 185 and follow it to Boat Landing Road. Turn left on Boat Landing Road to reach James R. Hines Boat Landing Park. The uppermost put-in is at the Tailwater Recreation Area below Barren River Lake Dam.

✧ **GAUGE** Call the Army Corps of Engineers' Barren River Lake Dam information hotline at 270-646-2122. It will tell you the water release from below the dam in cubic feet per second. The minimum reading should be 170 cfs.

GPS COORDINATES

ACCESS	LATITUDE	LONGITUDE
A	N36° 53.737'	W86° 7.810'
B	N36° 56.007'	W86° 12.242'
C	N36° 54.216'	W86° 14.084'
D	N36° 56.520'	W86° 15.330'
E	N36° 58.375'	W86° 22.941'
F	N37° 0.253'	W86° 25.006'
G	N37° 1.165'	W86° 23.587'

B Bowling Green to Green River

Class	I
Gauge	Phone
Level	Min. 400–Max. flood (cfs)
Gradient	0.7'
Scenery	C

54B **DESCRIPTION** Downstream from the mouth of Jennings Creek on the west side of Bowling Green, the Barren is a huge river, definitely navigable but not particularly appealing for paddlers. The river is runnable year-round, and is often broken by rather large, often named islands. Access between Bowling Green and the Green River is limited to a ramp below abandoned Lock 1 by Greencastle Road, on the east bank, and near Sallys Rock at the confluence of the Gasper River and the Barren River near KY 1435. Lock 1 is a hazard to navigation. Portage is strongly recommended!

✧ **SHUTTLE** To reach the landing just below the confluence of the Barren and Green Rivers,

take KY 231 North from Bowling Green toward Morgantown to KY 403. Turn right on KY 403 to reach the landing on the Green River in Woodbury. To reach the put-in on the west side of Bowling Green from Exit 26 on I-65, take KY 234 West in Bowling Green to KY 185. Turn right on KY 185 and follow it to Boat Landing Road. Turn left on Boat Landing Road to reach James R. Hines Boat Landing Park.

✧ **GAUGE** Call the Army Corps of Engineers' Barren River Lake Dam information hotline at 270-646-2122. It will tell you the water release from below the dam in cubic feet per second. Note: the river is runnable year-round at this point no matter the release schedule.

GPS COORDINATES

ACCESS	LATITUDE	LONGITUDE
G	N37° 1.165'	W86° 23.587'
H	N36° 56.007'	W86° 12.242'
I	N37° 5.415'	W86° 29.865'
J	N37° 5.094'	W86° 34.769'
K	N37° 11.030'	W86° 37.910'

Barren River: Bowling Green to Green River

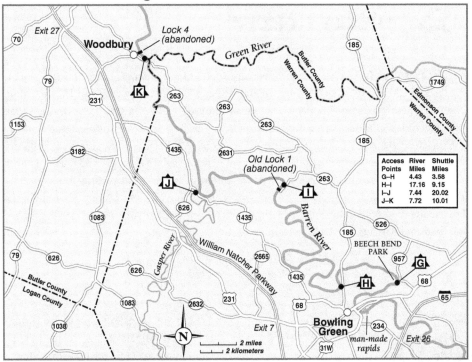

Access Points	River Miles	Shuttle Miles
G–H	4.43	3.58
H–I	17.16	9.15
I–J	7.44	20.02
J–K	7.72	10.01

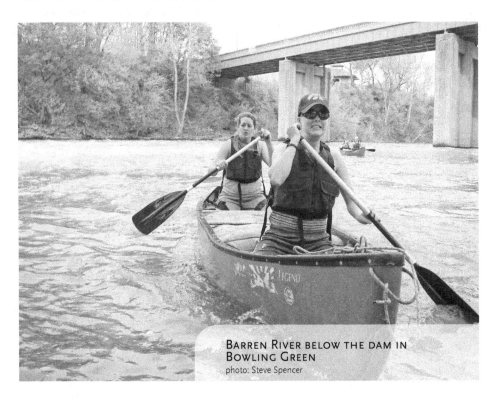

BARREN RIVER BELOW THE DAM IN
BOWLING GREEN
photo: Steve Spencer

55 DRAKES CREEK

◇ **OVERVIEW** Drakes Creek, along with its three feeder forks, comprises the drainage system for the area directly south of Bowling Green between US 31W on the west and US 231 on the east. Originating near the Tennessee border in Simpson and Allen Counties, Drakes Creek finally empties into the Barren River just outside Bowling Green. Running through deep, rolling farmland and wooded terrain, nearly the entire system provides excellent paddling opportunities. The West Fork and the Trammel Fork are suitable for paddling, as is Drakes Creek itself below the confluence of the forks. The width of the stream varies from 30 to 45 feet on the forks to 90 feet below the confluence. Deadfalls are not uncommon on the forks but usually do not block the entire stream. Access is excellent, with an unusually high number of paved county roads interlacing the entire area.

◇ **MAPS** DRAKE, ALLEN SPRINGS, POLKVILLE,
BOWLING GREEN SOUTH (USGS)

A Confluence to KY 234

Class	I+
Gauge	Web
Level	Min. 120–Max. flood (cfs)
Gradient	2.4'
Scenery	B

55A **DESCRIPTION** The put-in, Romanza Johnson County Park (CC), is just a bit above the confluence of West Fork and Trammel Fork on Trammel Fork. Drakes Creek below the confluence is runnable most of the year, although an occasional sandbar may have to be portaged during late summer and early fall. Islands, some of which are suitable for camping, can be found below the confluence. The width of the stream widens to 90 feet below the confluence. Shorter trips can be made using the US 231 bridge, where there is a boat ramp access (DD); the KY 2629 bridge (EE); and the water access off Cumberland Ridge Avenue near Middle Bridge Road (FF). Be careful at the KY 234 bridge (E) because traffic on this road has increased considerably over the past few years.

◇ **SHUTTLE** To reach the take-out from Exit 26 on I-65 in Bowling Green, take KY 234 South 0.5 mile to the bridge over Drakes Creek. To reach the put-in from the take-out, continue on KY 234 South for 2.6 miles. Turn right onto Hunts Lane and follow it 2.1 miles. Turn right onto Middle Bridge Road and go 0.1 mile. Turn left onto Roy Thomas Road and travel 0.6 mile. Turn left onto KY 872 and follow it 4.9 miles. Turn right onto Mount Lebanon Church Road and go 0.8 mile. Turn right onto Romanza Johnson Road to enter the park and access.

◇ **GAUGE** The USGS gauge is West Fork Drakes Creek near Franklin, KY. The minimum reading should be 120 cfs.

Drakes Creek

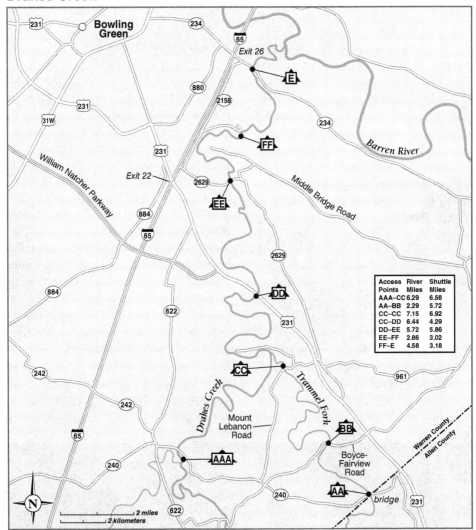

Access Points	River Miles	Shuttle Miles
AAA–CC	6.29	6.58
AA–BB	2.29	5.72
CC–CC	7.15	6.92
CC–DD	6.44	4.29
DD–EE	5.72	5.86
EE–FF	2.86	3.02
FF–E	4.58	3.18

B Upper Trammel Fork to Romanza Johnson County Park

Class	I+
Gauge	Web
Level	Min. 150–Max. flood (cfs)
Gradient	2.4'
Scenery	B

55B DESCRIPTION Running over a sand, rock, and clay bottom, the Trammel Fork of Drakes Creek follows a deep bed overhung by hardwoods. Watch for low trees and strainers at higher water levels. Boyce-Fairview Road (BB) offers an alternate access for a 2-mile trip from KY 240 or a 7-mile trip down to the confluence at Romanza Johnson County Park (CC).

◇ **SHUTTLE** To reach the take-out from Exit 20A on I-65, take the William Natcher Parkway for 2.4 miles, then merge onto US 231 South for 3.3 miles. Turn right onto Mount Lebanon Church Road and follow it 0.8 mile. Turn right onto Romanza Johnson Road and follow it to Romanza Johnson County Park and the take-out. To reach the put-in from the take-out, backtrack to US 231 and turn right. Take US 231 South for 3.4 miles, then turn right onto KY 240 West and follow it 1.1 miles to the bridge over Trammel Fork.

◇ **GAUGE** The USGS gauge is West Fork Drakes Creek near Franklin. The minimum reading should be 150 cfs.

≈≈≈

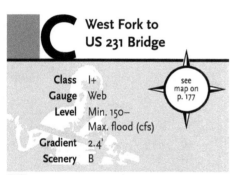

C West Fork to US 231 Bridge

Class	I+
Gauge	Web
Level	Min. 150– Max. flood (cfs)
Gradient	2.4'
Scenery	B

see map on p. 177

55C **DESCRIPTION** Banks vary in steepness and sometimes approach the appearance of a gorge on the West Fork where there are some vertical rock walls. Just enough riffles and current are found to make the paddling interesting. The West Fork averages 30–45 feet in width. Pools intersperse very simple (Class I+) shoals and rapids. The water quality is good, and very little trash is found near the stream. The trip could be shortened to 7 miles by pulling upstream at the confluence with Trammel Fork to Romanza Johnson Country Park (CC), which is on Trammel Fork.

◇ **SHUTTLE** To reach the take-out from Exit 20A on I-65, take the William Natcher Parkway for 2.4 miles, then merge onto US 231 South for 2.3 miles to the boat ramp on the right at the bridge over Drakes Creek. To reach the put-in from the take-out, continue 1 mile

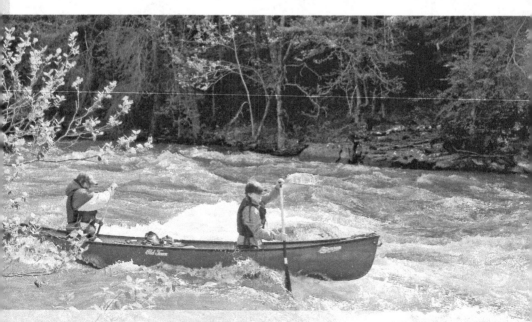

PADDLERS GASHING DOWN THE GASPER RIVER
photo: Steve Spencer

south on US 231, then turn right onto Mount Lebanon Church Road and follow it 2.8 miles. Make a slight left onto Mount Lebanon Road and travel 1 mile. Turn right onto KY 240 West and follow it 2.6 miles to the bridge over Drakes Creek.

❖ **GAUGE** The USGS gauge is West Fork Drakes Creek near Franklin. The minimum reading should be 150 cfs.

GPS Coordinates

ACCESS	LATITUDE	LONGITUDE
AA	N36° 49.634'	W86° 19.883'
AAA	N36° 50.359'	W86° 24.795'
BB	N36° 50.693'	W86° 20.945'
CC	N36° 52.282'	W86° 22.134'
DD	N36° 53.720'	W86° 22.850'
EE	N36° 56.093'	W86° 23.525'
FF	N36° 57.013'	W86° 23.258'
E	N36° 58.375'	W86° 22.941'

56 GASPER RIVER

❖ **OVERVIEW** The Gasper River is one of western Kentucky's most beautiful waterways. A tributary of the Barren River, the Gasper River drains the area between Russellville and Bowling Green. Runnable from mid-November to mid-May, the Gasper flows over a rock, sand, and clay bottom around medium-size boulders through a small gorge with steep, exposed rock walls rising almost vertically from the river's edge.

❖ **MAPS** SOUTH UNION, SUGAR GROVE, HADLEY (USGS)

Bucksville to Barren River

Class	I–II
Gauge	Visual, web
Level	Min. 220–
	Max. 500/flood (cfs)
Gradient	4.8'
Scenery	B

see map on p. 180

❖ **DESCRIPTION** The Gasper can be paddled from the Liberty Church Road bridge (A) to its mouth at the Barren River (G). Rated Class II, the Gasper sports a few interesting small rapids and a fairly swift current. Most of the river is very compact, with its width not exceeding 40 feet until just upstream of the KY 626 bridge (E), where the stream broadens to 60–80 feet, though Clear Fork Creek adds significant volume just above the KY 1083 bridge. The upper, narrower sections (above KY 626) are potentially dangerous at high water levels due to frequent strainers (deadfalls) and the lack of eddies. Access from intersecting bridges is not always easy, but it is possible, making runs from 3 to 11 miles possible. The access at the US 231 bridge (F) has improved.

❖ **SHUTTLE** To reach the lowest access point from Exit 7 on the William Natcher Parkway just west of Bowling Green, take US 231 North to KY 626. Turn right on KY 626 to reach KY 1435. Turn right on KY 1435 and pass over the Gasper River bridge; the take-out will be on the left, just upstream on the Barren River. To reach the uppermost access point from Bowling Green, take US 68 South to KY 1083. Turn right on KY 1083 West to reach KY 1038. Turn

Gasper River

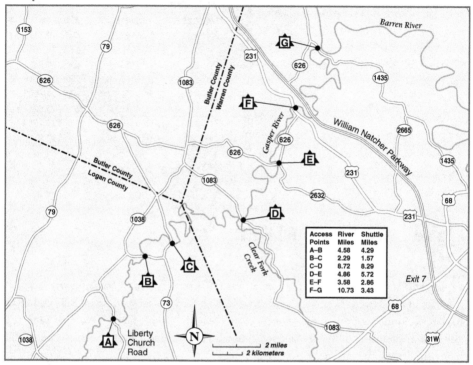

Access Points	River Miles	Shuttle Miles
A–B	4.58	4.29
B–C	2.29	1.57
C–D	8.72	8.29
D–E	4.86	5.72
E–F	3.58	2.86
F–G	10.73	3.43

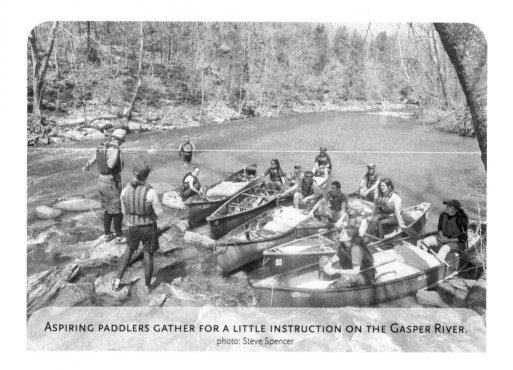

ASPIRING PADDLERS GATHER FOR A LITTLE INSTRUCTION ON THE GASPER RIVER.
photo: Steve Spencer

left on KY 1038 and follow it to Liberty Church Road. Turn left on Liberty Church Road to the Gasper River bridge.

✧ **GAUGE** The Gasper is generally high enough to be run from mid-November to mid-May and when the nearby Barren is high and muddy. An imperfect but helpful comparison gauge is West Fork Drakes Creek near Franklin. The minimum reading should be 220 cfs.

GPS COORDINATES

ACCESS	LATITUDE	LONGITUDE
A	N36° 56.211'	W86° 43.365'
B	N36° 58.253'	W86° 42.015'
C	N36° 58.682'	W86° 40.899'
D	N36° 59.437'	W86° 37.882'
E	N37° 1.335'	W86° 36.404'
F	N37° 3.186'	W86° 35.748'
G	N37° 1.165'	W86° 23.587'

57 LITTLE BARREN RIVER

✧ **OVERVIEW** The Little Barren River, with its east and south forks, drains most of Metcalfe County and the western portion of Green County before emptying into the Green River west of Greensburg. In the upper sections, both forks are runnable. The two forks are intimate and scenic, running between steep hills over rock and mud bottoms. Both forks average 30–40 feet in width. The Little Barren River opens up somewhat below the forks. Access is good, and navigational hazards are limited to deadfalls. Access below the confluence of the forks is fair to good (so rated because of a rather difficult access point at the KY 88 bridge). Deadfalls are the primary hazards to navigation.

✧ **MAPS** SULPHUR WELL, EAST FORK, CENTER (USGS)

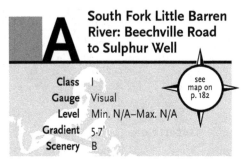

A South Fork Little Barren River: Beechville Road to Sulphur Well

Class	I
Gauge	Visual
Level	Min. N/A–Max. N/A
Gradient	5.7'
Scenery	B

see map on p. 182

57A **DESCRIPTION** The South Fork is partially spring fed and can be run from late October through June downstream of the Rockland Mills Road low-water bridge (A). A shorter run can be made by starting at the park in the historic hamlet of Sulphur Well (B). This section drains more farm country, thus is more prone to staining after heavy rains.

✧ **SHUTTLE** To reach the take-out from Edmonton, take US 68 North 9 miles, then turn left onto KY 70 West and follow it 1.5 miles to reach the access on the northeast side of the bridge. To reach the put-in from the take-out, continue on KY 70 West for 2 miles, then turn left on Rockland Mills Road and go 2.1 miles to the bridge over South Fork.

✧ **GAUGE** The first few riffles near Rockland Mills Road should give you an idea whether it is floatable. If the South Fork is too low, try the Little Barren from the fork's confluence.

Little Barren River

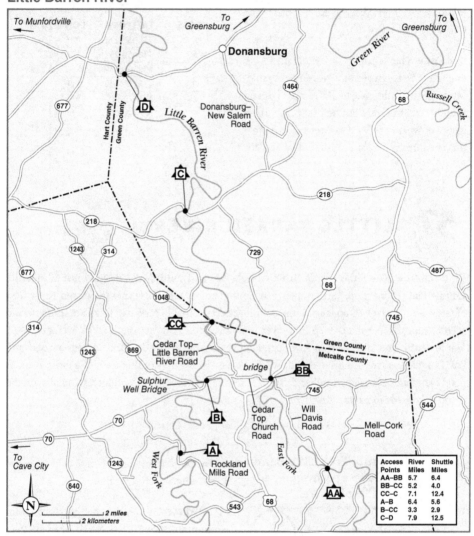

To Munfordville

To Greensburg

To Greensburg

Donansburg

Green River

Russell Creek

677

1464

68

D

Hart County

Green County

Little Barren River

Donansburg–
New Salem
Road

C

218

218

218

1243

314

729

487

677

68

1048

745

CC

Cedar Top–
Little Barren
River Road

Green County

Metcalfe County

1243

869

bridge

BB

Sulphur
Well Bridge

745

544

70

B

Cedar
Top
Church
Road

Will
Davis
Road

Mell–Cork
Road

70

West Fork

A

East Fork

AA

To
Cave City

1243

Rockland
Mills Road

640

543

68

N

2 miles

2 kilometers

Access Points	River Miles	Shuttle Miles
AA–BB	5.7	6.4
BB–CC	5.2	4.0
CC–C	7.1	12.4
A–B	6.4	5.6
B–CC	3.3	2.9
C–D	7.9	12.5

B
East Fork Little Barren River: Mell Cork Road to KY 745 Bridge

Class	I+
Gauge	Visual
Level	Min. N/A–Max. N/A
Gradient	9'
Scenery	B

57B **DESCRIPTION** The East Fork a more interesting run than the South Fork, with small rapids and ledges occurring frequently. The level of difficulty is Class I+. On average, the East Fork can be run from late fall through the spring below the Mell-Cork Road bridge (AA).

⬦ **SHUTTLE** To reach the take-out from Edmonton, take US 68 North 8.4 miles to the bridge over East Fork. To reach the put-in from the take-out, keep northeast on US 68 just a few feet, then turn right onto KY 745/ Mell Ridge Road and follow it 0.8 mile. Turn right onto Will Davis Road and go 2.6 miles. Turn right onto Mell Cork Road and follow it 200 feet to the bridge over the East Fork.

Little Barren River: Confluence of East Fork and South Fork to KY 88

Class	I+
Gauge	Visual
Level	Min. N/A–Max. N/A
Gradient	3.3'
Scenery	B

57C **DESCRIPTION** The valley deepens below the confluence of the two forks, with more exposed rock visible. The river widens to an average of 50–60 feet. Banks are 20 feet high here and generally steep. As the Little Barren approaches its mouth at the Green River, sand-bars become more numerous, and the steeper terrain of southern Green and northern Metcalfe Counties gives way to more gently rolling farm- and woodland. A shorter run can be made using KY 218 (C) as an access.

◇ GAUGE The water at the Mell-Cork bridge is a good indicator. If you can run this part, then you should make it all the way down.

◇ SHUTTLE From Greensburg, take KY 81 to KY 88. Turn left on KY 88 and follow it past the Green River to the Little Barren River. To reach the put-in, take KY 70 to Cedar Top Church Road (make sure to pick up Cedar Top Church Road west of where KY 70 and US 68 diverge). Turn right on Cedar Top Church Road, then quickly take a left on Cedar Top–Little Barren River Road to the confluence of the East Fork and South Fork.

◇ GAUGE There is no gauge. However, of the runs in the Little Barren River watershed, this section can be floated year-round, except for periods of extreme dryness.

GPS COORDINATES

ACCESS	LATITUDE	LONGITUDE	ACCESS	LATITUDE	LONGITUDE
AA	N37° 3.895'	W85° 34.180'	B	N37° 6.028'	W85° 38.053'
BB	N37° 6.069'	W85° 35.947'	C	N37° 10.204'	W85° 38.722'
CC	N37° 7.440'	W85° 37.908'	D	N37° 13.548'	W85° 40.649'
A	N37° 4.270'	W85° 38.856'			

58 NOLIN RIVER

◇ **OVERVIEW** The Nolin River winds out of the hilly farm country of Hardin County and flows south along the Grayson–Hart County line to empty into Nolin River Lake. Below the Nolin Dam in Edmonson County, the Nolin continues south to its confluence with the Green River in Mammoth Cave National Park. Because the stream is bordered without exception by private property, waterside camping is only recommended within the confines of Nolin River Lake and below the Nolin River Lake Dam within Mammoth Cave National Park.

◇ **MAPS** SONORA, SUMMIT, MILLERSTOWN, CUB RUN, NOLIN RESERVOIR, RHODA (USGS); MAMMOTH CAVE NATIONAL PARK MAP

A KY 1868 to Nolin River Lake

Class	I
Gauge	Visual
Level	Min. N/A–Max. N/A
Gradient	2.1'
Scenery	B

58A DESCRIPTION An attractive, tree-lined river averaging 35–50 feet wide, the Nolin flows between steep banks over a rock and mud bottom. Throughout the upper sections in Hardin County, the terrain is gently rolling with farms adjoining the river. South of Star Mills, the river valley deepens, with steep hills rising from time to time along the west bank. From this point to the headwaters of Nolin River Lake, the stream is interrupted four times by the remnants of dams from a once-flourishing mill industry. The Nolin River is runnable from late fall to mid-summer from KY 84 (D) to Wheelers Mill, near the KY 728 bridge. From Wheelers Mill to the headwaters of the lake, the Nolin is runnable year-round. Access for all varied runs above the lake is good. The uppermost access (A) is at Taylors Bend Park. Dangers in these upper sections include deadfalls, and, as mentioned, dams. All of the dams can be portaged without difficulty except at extremely high water levels.

With the exception of the dam at Star Mills (B), all of the dams are extremely dangerous and should not be run for any reason. At Star Mills, however, the dam has collapsed in two places, creating artificial Class II+ (borderline Class III) rapids. These rapids are runnable but should be scouted anew at every different water level. The last 24 miles of this section are on Nolin River Lake. It is 11 miles from KY 1868 to White Mills, 8 more miles to Spurrier, and 14 miles from Spurrier to the KY 1214 bridge. Nolin River Lake has numerous ramps and accesses but is heavy with powerboat traffic during the warm season.

◇ **SHUTTLE** To reach the take-out from US 31W in Bonnieville, take KY 728 West for 8.6 miles. Turn right onto KY 1214 and follow it 2.6 miles to the bridge over the Nolin River. To reach the put-in from the take-out, backtrack to US 31W in Bonnieville, turn left, and take 31W north for 13.4 miles. Turn left onto Gilead Church Road and follow it 2.8 miles. Turn left again onto KY 1136 and travel 0.5 mile. Take another left into Taylors Bend Park and an access point.

◇ **GAUGE** This is a look-and-see proposition. The upper Nolin is generally runnable from November to late June.

Nolin River: KY 1868 to Nolin River Lake

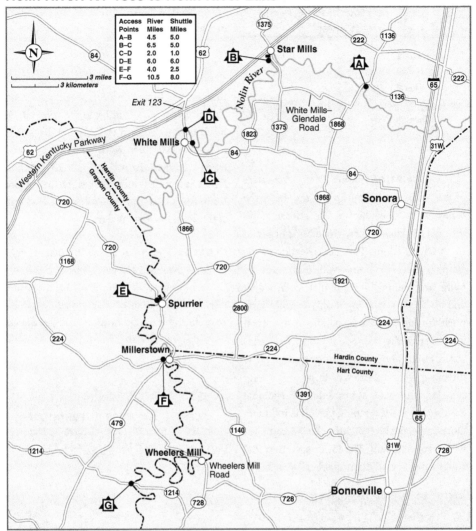

Access Points	River Miles	Shuttle Miles
A–B	4.5	5.0
B–C	6.5	5.0
C–D	2.0	1.0
D–E	6.0	6.0
E–F	4.0	2.5
F–G	10.5	8.0

GPS Coordinates

ACCESS	LATITUDE	LONGITUDE	ACCESS	LATITUDE	LONGITUDE
A	N37° 35.025'	W85° 54.987'	E	N37° 28.490'	W86° 3.303'
B	N37° 35.880'	W85° 58.760'	F	N37° 26.654'	W86° 3.041'
C	N37° 33.321'	W86° 1.913'	G	N37° 22.866'	W86° 4.335'
D	N37° 33.706'	W86° 2.142'			

B Nolin River Lake Dam to Houchins Ferry on Green River

Class	I
Gauge	Web
Level	250
Gradient	2.2'
Scenery	B+

58B DESCRIPTION From the tailwaters of the Nolin River Dam to the mouth of the Nolin at the Green River, the stream flows through the backcountry woodlands of Mammoth Cave National Park. This section of the Nolin is especially scenic with high, exposed bluffs and plentiful wildlife, particularly deer and ducks. This section is only 9 miles long (including an easy 2-mile paddle upstream on the Green to the take-out at Houchins Ferry) but affords some beautiful camping spots for those with a short way to go and a long time to get there. A Mammoth Cave National Park backcountry camping permit is required. Once again, the level of difficulty is Class I but with a good current. The lower section of the Nolin River is usually runnable all year but is entirely dependent on releases at the dam for adequate flow. Navigational hazards are limited to deadfalls. The average stream width is 50–80 feet. Access is good.

⟡ SHUTTLE To access the take-out from Brownsville, leave Main Street and take Houchins Ferry Road 1.6 miles to the take-out. To reach the put-in from the take-out, backtrack to Brownsville, turn right onto KY 259, and travel 7.3 miles. Turn right onto KY 728 and follow it 2 miles, then split right just before Nolin River Lake Dam. Descend and dead-end at the access below the dam.

⟡ GAUGE The Nolin below the dam is runnable year-round. However, check the Army Corps of Engineers Nolin River Lake website, then click on "Lake Levels," find Nolin River Lake, find the 6 a.m. outflow, and get the cfs release from the dam. The minimum should be 250 cfs.

GPS Coordinates

ACCESS	LATITUDE	LONGITUDE
H	N37° 16.430'	W86° 15.090'
I	N37° 12.160'	W86° 14.250'

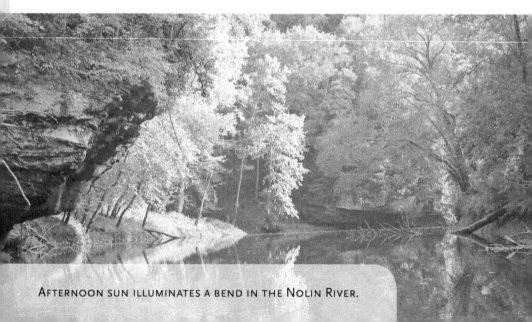

AFTERNOON SUN ILLUMINATES A BEND IN THE NOLIN RIVER.

Nolin River: Nolin River Lake Dam to Houchins Ferry on Green River

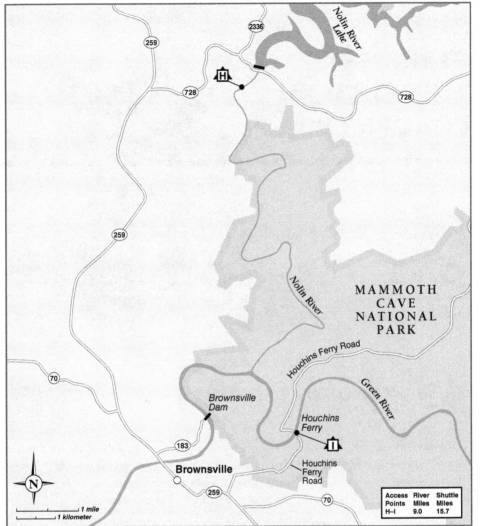

Access Points	River Miles	Shuttle Miles
H–I	9.0	15.7

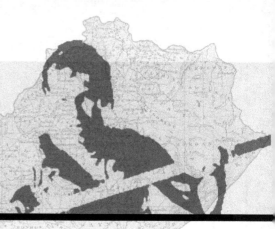

PART EIGHT
STREAMS OF THE WESTERN COAL FIELDS

59 TRADEWATER RIVER

◇ **OVERVIEW** Everyone in western Kentucky knows about the tragedy of the Tradewater River—that sterile, lifeless stream appropriated as a private sewer for the mining industry. The Tradewater River runs north from Christian County and empties into the Ohio River west of Sturgis. However, it's popularity as a paddler destination has increased of late.

◇ **MAPS** DAWSON SPRINGS, OLNEY, DALTON, PROVIDENCE, BLACKFORD, STURGIS, DEKOVEN (USGS)

KY 70 to Ohio River

Class	I
Gauge	Web
Level	Min. 130–Max. flood (cfs)
Gradient	0.7'
Scenery	C–

◇ **DESCRIPTION** Although the water here is almost devoid of life, the stream is nevertheless pleasing to the eye. An intimate river, with willow and hardwood completely shading the water, it winds through rolling farm and mining country. The Tradewater River is generally runnable most of the year downstream of the KY 293 bridge (B), although an occasional shallow may have to be portaged in late summer and early fall. The river channel is generally deep, thereby facilitating paddling, and it is not normally cluttered with deadfalls downstream of the KY 120 bridge (D). However, the river is more appealing further upstream.

Tradewater River

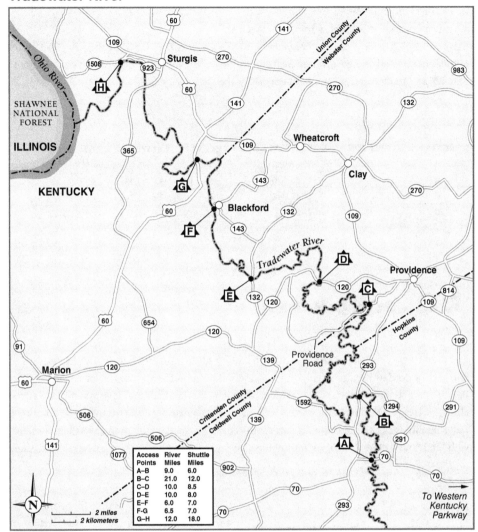

Access Points	River Miles	Shuttle Miles
A–B	9.0	6.0
B–C	21.0	12.0
C–D	10.0	8.5
D–E	10.0	8.0
E–F	6.0	7.0
F–G	6.5	7.0
G–H	12.0	18.0

The bottom and banks of the river are mud and vary markedly in their degree of slope. Cypress trees are abundant. The gradient is gentle, and current is moderate to slow. The river expands from 35 feet in width at the KY 293 bridge to around 110 feet near its mouth. Numerous access points allow for trips of varied lengths. Overnight paddler camping near the stream is possible at low water levels. Access on the Tradewater has greatly improved, serving as a model for other lesser visited Kentucky rivers. Boat ramps have been added at the Providence Road crossing (C), the KY 120 bridge (D), the KY 132 bridge (E), US 60 bridge (G), and off Old Providence Avenue in Sturgis (H).

✧ **SHUTTLE** To reach the take-out from downtown Sturgis, follow North Monroe Street/KY 365 south 1.6 miles to reach the bridge over the Tradewater River. To reach the put-in from the take-out, continue south on KY 365 for 8.5 miles. Turn right onto US 60 and follow it 1.6 miles. Turn left onto KY 654 and go 4.3 miles. Turn left onto KY 120 East and follow it 5.5 miles, then keep straight, joining KY 139. Stay with KY 139 for 3 miles, then turn left onto Webster Road and go 3 miles. Turn right onto KY 293 and travel 1.5 miles. Turn left onto

KY 70 East and follow it 1 mile to the bridge over the Tradewater River.

⬦ GAUGE The USGS gauge is Tradewater River at Olney. The minimum reading should be 130 cfs.

GPS COORDINATES

ACCESS	LATITUDE	LONGITUDE
A	N37° 16.505'	W87° 47.954'
B	N37° 19.050'	W87° 48.620'
C	N37° 22.851'	W87° 48.048'
D	N37° 23.790'	W87° 50.700'

ACCESS	LATITUDE	LONGITUDE
E	N37° 23.932'	W87° 54.299'
F	N37° 26.756'	W87° 56.283'
G	N37° 28.762'	W87° 57.204'
H	N37° 32.719'	W88° 1.173'

60 POND RIVER

⬦ OVERVIEW The Pond River is a main tributary of the Green River. Its headwaters are in northern Todd County, and its mouth is west of Calhoun on the McLean–Hopkins border. The Pond River and its tributaries, all of which are small, are the main drainage system for eastern Hopkins, western Muhlenberg, northern Christian, and northern Todd Counties. Although the water quality is not the best due to some mining discharge, the stream is nevertheless scenic, with birch and willow trees overhanging the water, and it has a well-defined, navigable channel.

⬦ MAPS MILLPORT, SACRAMENTO, CALHOUN (USGS)

KY 70 to Green River

Class	I
Gauge	Web
Level	Min. 170–Max. flood (cfs)
Gradient	0.8'
Scenery	C

⬦ DESCRIPTION The Pond River is generally runnable all year from the KY 70 bridge to its mouth, although occasional shallows may have to be portaged in late summer and early fall. The river is generally clear of deadfalls and debris, but some may be encountered

upstream of KY 85 bridge (B), particularly after spring flooding. At the intersection of KY 70 (A), the Pond River is about 25 feet wide. Moving north, it stays small (under 50 feet) up to within 10 miles of its mouth, where it broadens to 80–100 feet. The river flows through gently rolling, flat farmland and occasionally through some woodland and mining country. Its bottom is of mud with generally high, steep banks. Access has gotten better, especially at the KY 254 crossing and at the confluence with the Green River (D), where there are ramps. Current is slow, except at high water. Riverside areas for canoe

Pond River

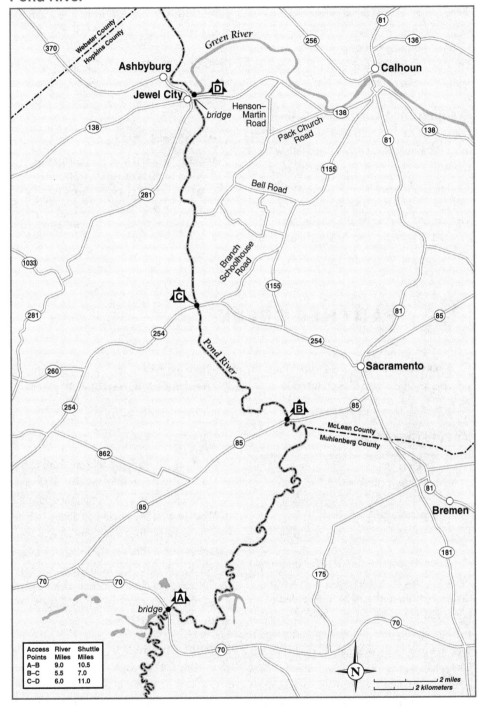

Access Points	River Miles	Shuttle Miles
A–B	9.0	10.5
B–C	5.5	7.0
C–D	6.0	11.0

camping are limited (even at low water) by the steep banks and the dense streamside vegetation. It is possible, however, to secure permission (in advance) to camp on the edge of the farm fields above the river if you contact the landowners in person.

✦ SHUTTLE To reach the take-out from Calhoun, take KY 81 South over the Green River. Turn right onto KY 138 West and follow it 5.8 miles to reach a boat ramp on the right, on the Green River, just above it's confluence with the Pond River. To reach the put-in from the take-out, backtrack to Calhoun, turn right onto KY 81 South, and follow it 10.5 miles.

Turn right onto KY 85 West and follow it 10.2 miles. Turn left onto KY 70 East to reach the bridge over the Pond River.

✦ GAUGE The USGS gauge is Pond River near Apex. The minimum reading should be 170 cfs.

GPS Coordinates

ACCESS	LATITUDE	LONGITUDE
A	N37° 19.042'	W87° 22.148'
B	N37° 23.685'	W87° 18.321'
C	N37° 26.520'	W87° 21.200'
D	N37° 31.655'	W87° 21.265'

61 PANTHER CREEK

✦ OVERVIEW Panther Creek constitutes the main drainage system for Daviess County and the area around Owensboro. The creek is paddleable but definitely not aesthetically pleasing.

✦ MAPS SUTHERLAND, PANTHER, CURDSVILLE (USGS)

KY 81 to Green River

Class	I
Gauge	Visual, web
Level	Min. 95–Max. flood (cfs)
Gradient	0.6'
Scenery	D

✦ DESCRIPTION At the KY 81 bridge (A) Panther Creek is narrow, resembles a dredged drainage ditch, and has been denuded of all but scrub vegetation 15 feet from its banks, presumably for the purpose of terracing. It soon returns to its original channel, but has been channelized downstream where it was extremely winding. The Panther runs through flat farmland. Its banks and bottom are of mud, steep, and 6–15 feet high. Water quality is poor. Access from intersecting bridges is not difficult.

✦ SHUTTLE To reach the take-out from Exit 11 on US 60 Bypass on the west side of Owensboro, take KY 81 west 0.7 mile, then join KY 56 West in a traffic circle and follow KY 56 West for 6 miles. Turn right onto KY 456 West and follow it 2.6 miles to the bridge over Panther Creek. To reach the put-in from the take-out, backtrack to the traffic circle at KY 81 and KY 56, then take KY 81 south 4.5 miles to the bridge over Panther Creek.

✦ GAUGE The creek is generally runnable from late fall through late spring. However, a helpful gauge is South Fork Panther Creek near Whitesville, KY. If it is running at or above normal from late fall through spring, you should have favorable water levels.

Panther Creek

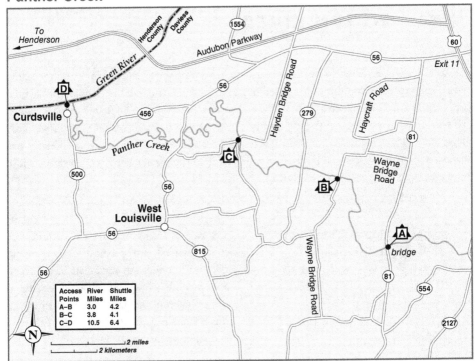

GPS Coordinates

ACCESS	LATITUDE	LONGITUDE	ACCESS	LATITUDE	LONGITUDE
A	N37° 41.395'	W87° 11.442'	C	N37° 43.608'	W87° 15.375'
B	N37° 42.800'	W87° 12.749'	D	N37° 31.655'	W87° 21.265'

62 ROUGH RIVER

✧ **OVERVIEW** The Rough River is not very rough but extremely paddleable. Running east to west over a rock bottom through wooded hill country and farmland, the Rough River is typically high banked and shaded with willow and various hardwoods. The Rough can be paddled all year from the tailwater of the Rough River Lake Dam to its mouth at the Green River near Livermore. Water quality is generally fair to good. Lateral erosion along the steep banks has exposed many tree roots and has caused a substantial number of deadfalls. The river's width averages from 50 to 70 feet throughout.

✧ **MAPS** McDaniels, Falls of Rough, Olaton, Dundee, Horton, Equality (USGS)

A Rough River Dam to Dundee

Class	I (II)
Gauge	Web
Level	Min. 165–Max. flood (cfs)
Gradient	1.4'
Scenery	B

62A **DESCRIPTION** The dam at Rough River Lake is being worked on, temporarily closing the tailwater access. Contact the Corps of Engineers office at 270-257-2061 before attempting to put in at the dam. Additionally, the Corps is establishing paddling trails on Rough River Lake, a boon for flatwater paddlers. On the Rough River, the most scenic sections are from the tailwater to Falls of the Rough, and from Falls of the Rough to the KY 54 bridge. Both of these sections sport some minor (Class I+) rapids, ripples, and shoals and occasional bluffs. The take-out at the KY 110 bridge (B) requires a major uphill pull. The land around the 7-foot dam at Falls of the Rough and old stores and buildings of the Falls of Rough community are now part of a golf course and resort. Ask for permission at the resort entrance station before portaging around the dam at Falls of Rough or using the

area as a put-in or take-out. The dam itself is considered extremely dangerous and should not be run under any circumstances. Several access points allow trips of varied lengths. It is 5 miles from the dam to Falls of Rough, 8 miles from Falls of Rough to Hite Falls (C), and 10 miles farther to Dundee (F).

✧ **SHUTTLE** The take-out is located at the bridge over the Rough River on KY 69, just north of the town of Dundee. To reach the put-in from the take-out, continue north on KY 69 for 2.5 miles, then turn right onto Narrows Road and follow it 0.4 mile to veer left onto Railroad Bed Road; follow Railroad Bed Road 2.1 miles to Barretts Road. Turn right onto Barretts Road and follow it 0.4 mile. Turn left onto Bud Baughn Road and follow it 0.9 mile. Turn right onto KY 54 and go 4.4 miles. Turn left onto KY 110 and travel 8.2 miles. Turn left onto KY 79 North and follow it 1.7 miles to turn left into the Tailwater Recreation Area below Rough River Lake Dam and an access.

✧ **GAUGE** The Rough below the dam is runnable year-round. Check the Army Corps of Engineers Rough River Lake website, then click "Lake Levels," then find the 6 a.m. outflow to get an idea of the cfs release from the dam.

Rough River: Rough River Dam to Dundee

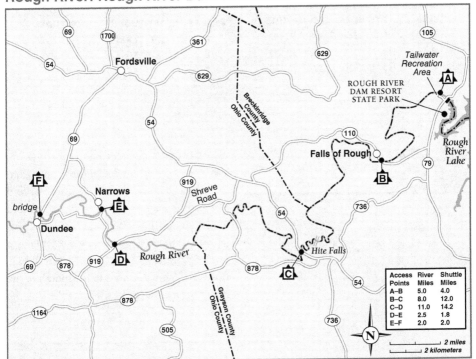

Access Points	River Miles	Shuttle Miles
A–B	5.0	4.0
B–C	8.0	12.0
C–D	11.0	14.2
D–E	2.5	1.8
E–F	2.0	2.0

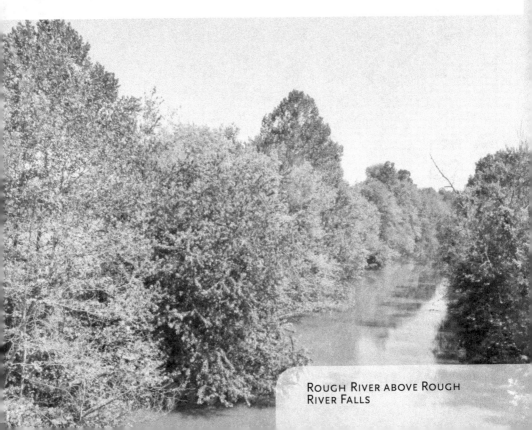

ROUGH RIVER ABOVE ROUGH RIVER FALLS

GPS Coordinates

ACCESS	LATITUDE	LONGITUDE	ACCESS	LATITUDE	LONGITUDE
A	N37° 37.345'	W86° 30.302'	D	N37° 32.828'	W86° 43.265'
B	N37° 35.272'	W86° 32.649'	E	N37° 33.906'	W86° 43.806'
C	N37° 32.530'	W86° 35.845'	F	N37° 33.777'	W86° 46.254'

B Dundee to Green River

Class	I
Gauge	Web
Level	Min. 190–Max. flood (cfs)
Gradient	0.6'
Scenery	C+

62B **DESCRIPTION** Moving farther downstream, access is limited downstream from the public boat ramp just west of Hartford (I), requiring an 18-mile run from Hartford to Livermore (J). Shorter floats are much easier near Dundee (F), including a 7.5-mile trip from Sunnydale Road (G) to Combs Bridge Road (H). From Hartford to the mouth of the Rough near Livermore, silver maples line the

Rough River: Dundee to Green River

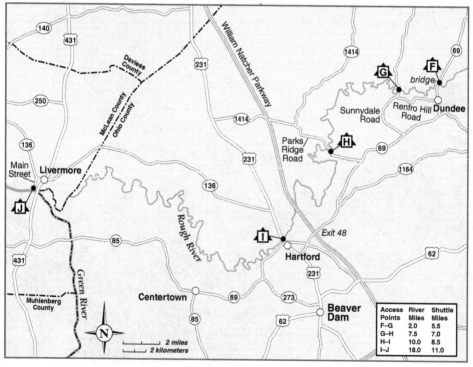

Access Points	River Miles	Shuttle Miles
F–G	2.0	5.5
G–H	7.5	7.0
H–I	10.0	8.5
I–J	18.0	11.0

watercourse. Watch out for and portage around the abandoned U.S. Army Corps of Engineers lock a few miles upstream of Livermore.

◇ SHUTTLE To reach the take-out in Livermore from Exit 48 on William Natcher Parkway, take KY 69 to Hartford. Turn right and head north on US 231 to KY 136. Turn left on KY 136 and follow it to US 431. Turn left and take US 431 South to Third Street. Turn right on Third Street, then turn left on Main Street, which leads to a boat ramp on the Green River just below the confluence with the Rough River. To reach the put-in from Exit 48 on Natcher Parkway, take KY 69 North to Dundee and the bridge over Rough River.

◇ GAUGE The Rough below the dam is runnable year-round. However, check the Army Corps of Engineers Rough River Lake website, click "Lake Levels," then find the 6 a.m. outflow to get an idea of the cfs release from the dam.

GPS COORDINATES

ACCESS	LATITUDE	LONGITUDE
F	N37° 33.777'	W86° 46.254'
G	N37° 33.456'	W86° 48.455'
H	N37° 30.889'	W86° 52.089'
I	N37° 27.186'	W86° 54.639'
J	N37° 33.906'	W86° 43.806'

63 MUD RIVER

◇ OVERVIEW The Mud River is an uninspiring stream originating near Russellville and running north over a mud bottom to empty into the Green River at Rochester. It is runnable from late fall to midsummer from the KY 949 bridge to its mouth.

◇ MAPS DUNMOR, ROCHESTER (USGS)

KY 949 to Rochester

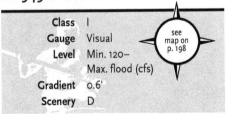

Class	I
Gauge	Visual
Level	Min. 120–
	Max. flood (cfs)
Gradient	0.6'
Scenery	D

see map on p. 198

◇ DESCRIPTION Access is good at bridge crossings and at the mouth but almost totally lacking in between. The Mud River runs primarily through hilly farmland. Banks are well vegetated and tree lined, but the water quality is poor due to mining waste discharge. Its width varies markedly from about 35 feet at

the KY 949 bridge, where there is a boat ramp (A), to almost 100 feet upstream of the KY 70 bridge. Deadfalls and some trash are in evidence on the narrower upstream sections.

◇ SHUTTLE To reach the lower access from Exit 28 on William Natcher Parkway, take KY 70 West to KY 2263. Turn right on KY 2263, then immediately turn left into the Rochester boat ramp on the Green River. To reach the upper access from Exit 28 on William Natcher Parkway, take KY 70 West to KY 106. Turn left on KY 106 to KY 949. Turn right on KY 949 and follow it to the bridge and ramp over Mud River.

Mud River

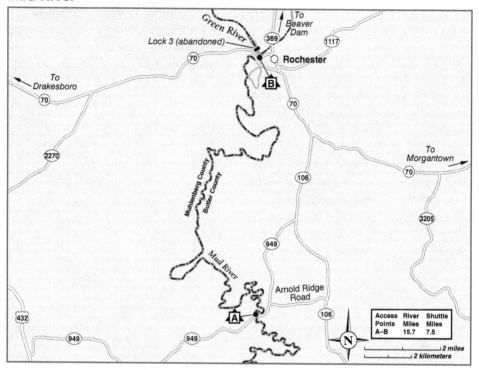

⟡ **GAUGE** Look to run the Mud from mid-November to early July or when the Green River is high.

GPS COORDINATES

ACCESS	LATITUDE	LONGITUDE
A	N37° 7.390'	W86° 54.028'
B	N37° 12.676'	W86° 53.969'

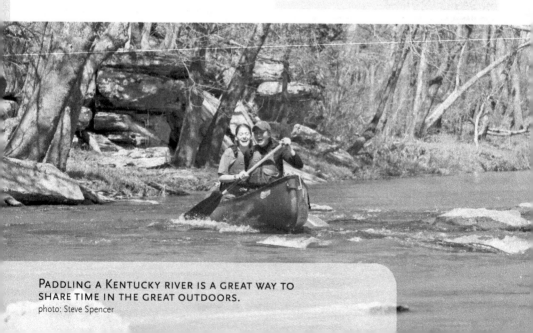

PADDLING A KENTUCKY RIVER IS A GREAT WAY TO SHARE TIME IN THE GREAT OUTDOORS.
photo: Steve Spencer

64 GREEN RIVER FROM HOUCHINS FERRY TO THE OHIO RIVER

◇ **OVERVIEW** This long, 185-mile section of the Green River is runnable all year, and access is plentiful, but unfortunately so are powerboats, barges, locks, and dams. In short, the lower Green River is one of Kentucky's primary commercial waterways and is not consistently appealing to paddlers. (Note: the upstream sections of the Green River are found in "Part Seven: Headwaters of the Green River.")

◇ **MAPS** RHODA, BROWNSVILLE, REEDYVILLE, RIVERSIDE, MORGANTOWN, FLENER, CROMWELL, SOUTH HILL, ROCHESTER, PARADISE, CENTRAL CITY EAST, CENTRAL CITY WEST, EQUALITY, LIVERMORE, GLENVILLE, CALHOUN, BEECH GROVE, DELAWARE, CURDSVILLE, REED, SPOTTSVILLE, NEWBURGH (USGS)

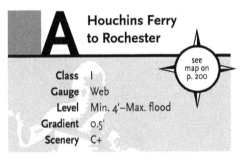

A Houchins Ferry to Rochester

see map on p. 200

Class	I
Gauge	Web
Level	Min. 4'–Max. flood
Gradient	0.5'
Scenery	C+

64A **DESCRIPTION** From Houchins Ferry, the Green River broadens considerably (increasing in volume) at its confluence with the Nolin River. Two miles farther downstream is the Brownsville Dam, a difficult portage at the old Lock 6. Old Lock 5 at Naker and old Lock 4 at Woodbury have been abandoned but nevertheless remain a danger to navigation. Portages are a must! From the dam to the mouth of the Barren River, the scenery remains pleasant, with farms and wooded hills. It is 35 miles from Houchins Ferry to Woodbury, 6 miles farther to Morgantown, and 37 miles from Morgantown to Rochester.

◇ **SHUTTLE** To reach the take-out from Exit 58 on the Western Kentucky Parkway, take US 431 South to KY 70. Turn left onto KY 70 and follow it east to the bridge over the Mud River. Turn left onto Russellville Street to reach a boat ramp on the Green River above old Lock 3. To reach the put-in from the take-out, continue east on KY 70 for 14 miles. Turn left onto US 231 and follow it 1.8 miles. Turn right onto KY 79 North and follow it 0.9 mile. Turn right onto KY 70 and follow it east 26 miles. Turn right onto KY 259 and follow it into Brownsville. Turn left onto Houchins Ferry Road and follow it 1.6 miles to the put-in.

◇ **GAUGE** The USGS gauge is Green River/ Lock 6 at Brownsville. The minimum reading should be 4 feet. This part of the Green is runnable year-round.

GPS COORDINATES

ACCESS	LATITUDE	LONGITUDE
Q	N37° 11.781'	W86° 16.559'
R	N37° 10.732'	W86° 21.663'
S	N37° 10.235'	W86° 23.912'
T	N37° 10.100'	W86° 23.940'
U	N37° 9.255'	W86° 24.509'
V	N37° 11.026'	W86° 37.905'
W	N37° 14.590'	W86° 41.295'
X	N37° 19.404'	W86° 46.453'
Y	N37° 15.600'	W86° 46.510'
Z	N37° 13.700'	W86° 46.777'
AA	N37° 12.676'	W86° 53.969'
BB	N37° 12.952'	W86° 54.189'

Green River: Houchins Ferry to Rochester

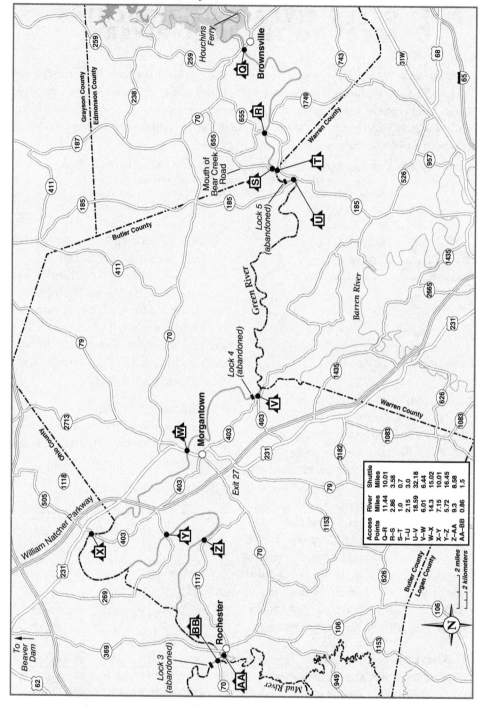

Access Points	River Miles	Shuttle Miles
Q–R	11.44	10.01
R–S	2.86	3.58
S–T	1.0	0.7
T–U	2.15	3.0
U–V	18.59	32.18
V–W	6.01	6.44
W–X	14.3	15.02
X–Y	7.15	10.01
Y–Z	5.72	16.45
Z–AA	9.3	8.58
AA–BB	0.86	1.5

B Rochester to Mouth of Pond River

Class I
Gauge Web
Level Min. 340–Max. flood (cfs)
Gradient 0.4'
Scenery C+

64B DESCRIPTION Old Lock 3 at Rochester, just above the put-in for this section, is abandoned. Put your boat in well below the flow. In this stretch, pleasure boaters constitute the majority of river traffic. As on any big river, the vistas are panoramic (if not often changing), access is excellent by virtue of the many ramps and marinas, and countless trip possibilities exist. It is 26 miles from Rochester to Central City, 17 miles from Central City to Livermore, 10 miles from Livermore to Calhoun, and 10 more miles to the mouth of the Pond River.

◇ SHUTTLE To reach the take-out from Exit 58 on the Western Kentucky Parkway, take US 431 North for 15.5 miles to join KY 138 West. Follow KY 138 West for 15 miles to the boat ramp on the right just before the bridge over the Pond River. To reach the Rochester put-in from Exit 58 on the Western Kentucky Parkway, take US 431 South to KY 70. Turn left on KY 70 and follow it east to KY 2263 and the bridge over Mud River. Look for a gravel road leading left to Muhlenburg County Park and boat ramp below old Lock 3. The county park and boat ramp are before KY 2263 and the bridge over Mud River. Do not put in at Rochester boat ramp, as this will be above old Lock 3.

Green River: Rochester to Mouth of Pond River

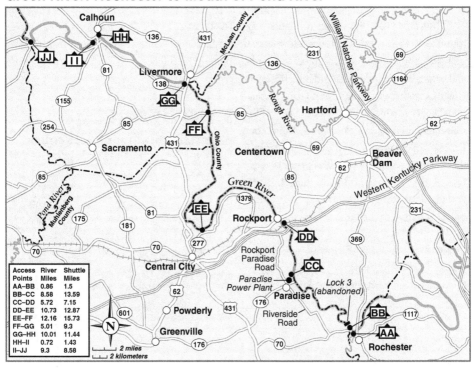

Access Points	River Miles	Shuttle Miles
AA–BB	0.86	1.5
BB–CC	8.58	13.59
CC–DD	5.72	7.15
DD–EE	10.73	12.87
EE–FF	12.16	15.73
FF–GG	5.01	9.3
GG–HH	10.01	11.44
HH–II	0.72	1.43
II–JJ	9.3	8.58

GAUGE The USGS gauge is Green River at Livermore. The minimum reading should be 5 feet. This part of the Green is runnable year-round.

GPS COORDINATES

ACCESS	LATITUDE	LONGITUDE	ACCESS	LATITUDE	LONGITUDE
AA	N37° 12.676'	W86° 53.969'	FF	N37° 27.154'	W87° 6.200'
BB	N37° 12.952'	W86° 54.189'	GG	N37° 33.906'	W86° 43.806'
CC	N37° 16.401'	W86° 59.099'	HH	N37° 32.150'	W87° 15.466'
DD	N37° 19.862'	W86° 59.829'	II	N37° 31.681'	W87° 15.986'
EE	N37° 19.424'	W87° 6.746'	JJ	N37° 31.655'	W87° 21.265'

C Mouth of Pond River to Ohio River

Class	I
Gauge	Web
Level	Min. 6'–Max. flood
Gradient	0.4'
Scenery	C

64C **DESCRIPTION** The river, runnable year-round down here, once belonged to the coal industry. But although coal tipples, rail yards, and barges are frequently in evidence, the lower Green is not totally lacking in charm. Navigational hazards consist almost exclusively of the well-marked locks and dams. Lock 2 and Lock 1 are still in operation. Exercise caution around these facilities. The Spottsville take-out is above Lock 1. It is 19 miles from the mouth of the Pond River to Rangers Landing on KY 136 and 23 miles farther to the Ohio River.

SHUTTLE To reach the lowest access from Exit 81 on Breathitt Parkway, take US 60 East to Spottsville. Turn right on Spring Street just before the bridge over Green River and stay left with KY 2243 to turn left on Olhend-Spottsville Road and reach the Joe Pruden Boat Ramp at Willow Creek on the Green River one-half mile above Lock 1. To reach the upper access from Exit 54 on Breathitt Parkway, take KY 138 East to the bridge over the Pond River just above the Green River.

GAUGE The USGS gauge is Green River at Lock 2 at Calhoun. The minimum reading should be 6 feet.

GPS COORDINATES

ACCESS	LATITUDE	LONGITUDE
JJ	N37° 31.655'	W87° 21.265'
KK	N37° 35.401'	W87° 24.253'
LL	N37° 37.407'	W87° 29.915'
MM	N37° 40.075'	W87° 27.509'
NN	N37° 31.655'	W87° 21.265'
OO	N37° 48.227'	W87° 22.851'
PP	N37° 51.295'	W87° 24.495'
QQ	N37° 53.720'	W87° 27.780'

Green River: Mouth of Pond River to Ohio River

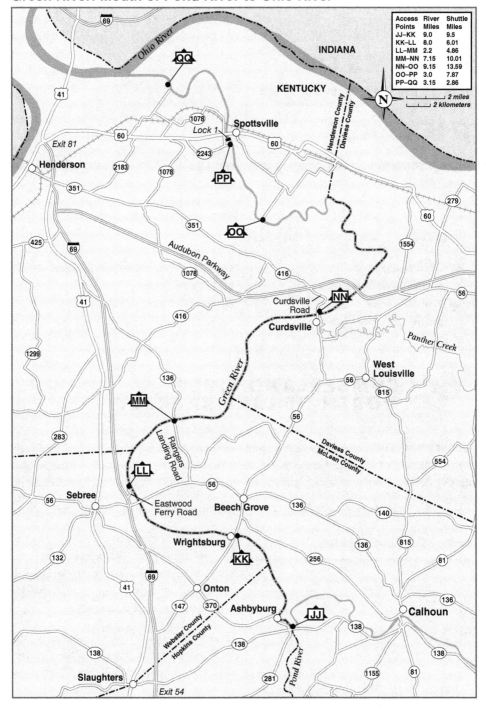

Access Points	River Miles	Shuttle Miles
JJ–KK	9.0	9.5
KK–LL	8.0	6.01
LL–MM	2.2	4.86
MM–NN	7.15	10.01
NN–OO	9.15	13.59
OO–PP	3.0	7.87
PP–QQ	3.15	2.86

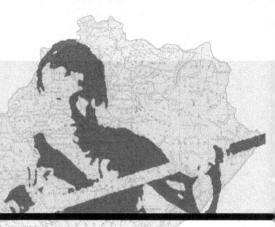

PART NINE
STREAMS OF LAND BETWEEN THE LAKES

65 CUMBERLAND RIVER NORTH OF LAKE BARKLEY

✧ **OVERVIEW** This section of the Cumberland River flows northwest from the tailwaters of Barkley Dam through Livingston County to the Ohio River. Pleasant but decidedly unspectacular, the Cumberland River makes long, graceful curves through the hilly farmland east of Paducah.

✧ **MAPS** Grand Rivers, Dycusburg, Burna, Smithland (USGS)

Barkley Dam to Ohio River

Class	I
Gauge	Phone
Level	Min. N/A–Max. N/A
Gradient	0.4'
Scenery	C+

✧ **DESCRIPTION** Trees (primarily willow) line the riverside but do not consistently obstruct the paddler's view of surrounding farms, small towns, and occasional businesses. The average width below the dam is 240 feet. Powerboats of all sizes are common. This section of the Cumberland is runnable all year. Access is good. The level of difficulty is Class I, with no navigational dangers except powerboats.

✧ **SHUTTLE** The take-out is located at the boat ramp at the confluence of the Cumberland River and the Ohio River in Smithland, off Riverfront Drive. To reach the put-in from the take-out, take KY 453 South out of Smithland for 11 miles, then join US 62 East for 2.2 miles. Turn right at the signed turn for the boat

Cumberland River North of Lake Barkley and Tennessee River North of Kentucky Lake

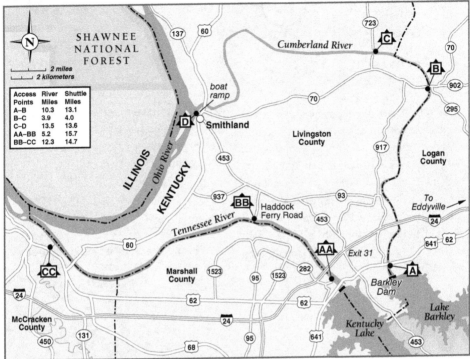

SHAWNEE NATIONAL FOREST

Access Points	River Miles	Shuttle Miles
A–B	10.3	13.1
B–C	3.9	4.0
C–D	13.5	13.6
AA–BB	5.2	15.7
BB–CC	12.3	14.7

ramp, then turn right again at the signed turn to reach the ramp below Lake Barkley Dam.

GAUGE Call the TVA Lake Information Line at 800-238-2264, then press 4, then 40, to get the latest water release from Barkley Lake Dam in cfs.

GPS Coordinates

ACCESS	LATITUDE	LONGITUDE
A	N37° 1.719'	W88° 13.558'
B	N37° 9.510'	W88° 11.301'
C	N37° 11.149'	W88° 14.380'
D	N37° 8.530'	W88° 24.450'

66 TENNESSEE RIVER NORTH OF KENTUCKY LAKE

OVERVIEW This 16-mile section of the Tennessee River flowing north along the southern boundary of Livingston County is all that is left of the beautiful Tennessee River in the state of Kentucky.

MAPS CALVERT CITY, LITTLE CYPRESS, PADUCAH EAST (USGS)

Kentucky Dam to Mouth of Clarks River

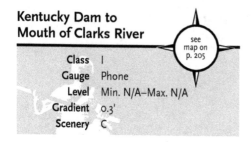

see map on p. 205

Class	I
Gauge	Phone
Level	Min. N/A–Max. N/A
Gradient	0.3'
Scenery	C

◇ **DESCRIPTION** Averaging 200–250 feet in width, this section of the Tennessee accommodates almost continuous commercial traffic. Scenery is similar to that of the Cumberland River below Barkley Dam except that the river valley here is somewhat deeper. Runnable all year, access is good where it exists. The level of difficulty is Class I with power craft, particularly barges, constituting the major danger to paddlers.

◇ **SHUTTLE** To reach the take-out at the mouth of the Clarks River from Exit 16 on I-24, take US 68 West to US 62. Turn left and take US 62 West to Clarks River boat ramp below bridge over Clarks River. To reach the put-in below Kentucky Dam from Exit 27 on I-24, take US 62 East to KY 282. Take KY 282 West to Cirrito Lane. Turn right on Cirrito Lane to reach a boat ramp on the river.

◇ **GAUGE** Runnable year-round. Call the TVA Lake Information Line at 800-238-2264, then press 4, then 33 to get the water release from Kentucky Lake Dam in cfs.

GPS COORDINATES

ACCESS	LATITUDE	LONGITUDE
AA	N37° 1.170'	W88° 16.810'
BB	N37° 3.830'	W88° 21.220'
CC	N37° 2.626'	W88° 32.829'

67 MUDDY FORK OF THE LITTLE RIVER

◇ **OVERVIEW** The Muddy Fork of the Little River originates in western Christian County and flows west to drain northern Trigg County before emptying into Lake Barkley.

◇ **MAPS** Cobb, Cadiz, Lamasco, Canton (USGS)

Adams Mill Road Bridge to Lake Barkley

Class	I+
Gauge	Web
Level	Min. 220–Max. flood (cfs)
Gradient	0.7'
Scenery	B–

◇ **DESCRIPTION** The Muddy Fork (not to be confused with the Mud River) is in many ways an inviting, intimate stream. The banks are steep, profusely shaded with tall hardwoods, and from time to time exposed rock is visible at water's edge. Averaging 35 feet in width, the Muddy Fork can be run from late fall to midsummer downstream of the Adams Mill bridge, and its proximity to Lake Barkley makes paddler camping possible. Scenery streamside consists of rolling farm- and

Little River and
Muddy Fork of the Little River

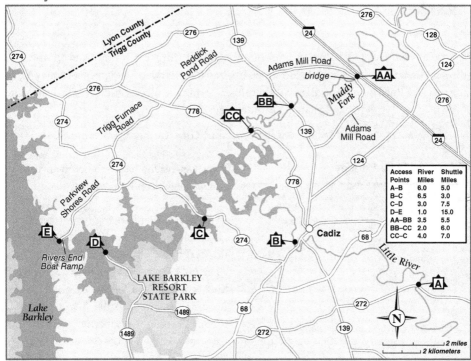

Access Points	River Miles	Shuttle Miles
A–B	6.0	5.0
B–C	6.5	3.0
C–D	3.0	7.5
D–E	1.0	15.0
AA–BB	3.5	5.5
BB–CC	2.0	6.0
CC–C	4.0	7.0

woodland (which you cannot see except in winter because of the dense foliage along the banks). The level of difficulty is Class I throughout with deadfalls (and some flash flooding in the upper sections) being the only hazards to navigation. Steep banks make access fair to difficult.

✧ **SHUTTLE** To reach the take-out from Cadiz, take Main Street south 1.1 miles. Turn right onto KY 274 North and follow it 4.1 miles, crossing the Little River embayment of Lake Barkley, and then coming to the boat ramp on the right just after the bridge over the embayment. To reach the put-in from the take-out, return to Cadiz and take KY 139 North for 2.4 miles. Turn right onto Adams Mill Road and go 2.8 miles to the bridge over the Muddy Fork.

✧ **GAUGE** The USGS gauge is Little River near Cadiz. The minimum reading should be 220 cfs.

GPS COORDINATES

ACCESS	LATITUDE	LONGITUDE
AA	N36° 55.580'	W87° 48.508'
BB	N36° 54.832'	W87° 50.658'
CC	N36° 54.255'	W87° 51.968'
A	N36° 50.457'	W87° 46.626'
B	N36° 51.505'	W87° 50.578'
C	N36° 52.101'	W87° 53.373'
D	N36° 51.220'	W87° 56.570'
E	N36° 51.548'	W87° 58.052'

68 LITTLE RIVER

✧ **OVERVIEW** The Little River originates in southern Christian County and flows north through Cadiz in Trigg County before emptying into Lake Barkley. The upper section is winding and tree lined with some giant, virgin timber. Terrain is hilly and rolling. The banks and bed are of mud with thick vegetation near the river's edge.

✧ **MAPS** ROARING SPRING, CALEDONIA, CADIZ, COBB, LAMASCO, CANTON (USGS)

KY 272 to Lake Barkley

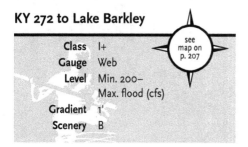

Class	I+
Gauge	Web
Level	Min. 200– Max. flood (cfs)
Gradient	1'
Scenery	B

see map on p. 207

✧ **DESCRIPTION** A good paddle-camping run, the Little River is runnable below the KY 272 bridge to Cadiz (there is a boat ramp at the US 68 bridge) from November to mid-July and from Cadiz to Lake Barkley all year long. Access is good. Some deadfalls, a fallen bridge, and a small 1-foot dam pose the only difficulties to navigation. From Cadiz downstream, there is no current due to the backed-up lake pool. It is 6 miles from KY 272 to the slack pool in Cadiz. The river broadens from 45 feet in the upper stretches to 60–75 feet below Cadiz. Surrounding hillsides are steeper with some exposed rock visible. There are no real hazards to navigation below Cadiz except an occasional gusty wind coming off the lake. Access is excellent, especially the Army Corps of Engineers ramps and Lake Barkley State Park marina. Runs on the Little

River can readily be combined with trips of various lengths on Lake Barkley.

✧ **SHUTTLE** To reach the lowest access on Lake Barkley from Exit 65 on I-24, take US 68 West to US 68 Business to KY 274. Turn right on KY 274 and follow it to Parkview Shores Road. Turn left on Parkview Shores Road and follow it to the Rivers End Boat Ramp. To reach the uppermost access from Exit 65 on I-24, take US 68 West to KY 139. Turn left on KY 139 and follow it to KY 272. Turn left and take KY 272 East to the bridge over Little River.

✧ **GAUGE** The USGS gauge is Little River near Cadiz. Minimum reading should be 200 cfs.

GPS COORDINATES

ACCESS	LATITUDE	LONGITUDE
AA	N36° 55.580'	W87° 48.508'
BB	N36° 54.832'	W87° 50.658'
CC	N36° 54.255'	W87° 51.968'
A	N36° 50.457'	W87° 46.626'
B	N36° 51.505'	W87° 50.578'
C	N36° 52.101'	W87° 53.373'
D	N36° 51.220'	W87° 56.570'
E	N36° 51.548'	W87° 58.052'

69 LAND BETWEEN THE LAKES PADDLE ROUTE

✧ **OVERVIEW** Look at a map of the United States, then focus on middle America. Try to find any body of water with 300 miles of undeveloped shoreline. Only one place offers such a shoreline—Land Between the Lakes (LBL). Here paddlers in both canoes and sea kayaks can travel along the bays and bluffs of Kentucky Lake and Lake Barkley. Adventurous paddlers will circumnavigate the long peninsula of the LBL, making nearly a loop separated by less than 10 miles of land. Paddlers can go for days without backtracking and still end up fairly close to their car and point of origin. The 85 miles is the shortest possible route of an LBL peninsula circumnavigation without exploring bays or making any side trips. A look at the map will show that this route can be extended by many miles and from 5 days to over 2 weeks. If not camping at campgrounds, paddlers must purchase a backcountry camping permit, available at the LBL visitor centers and online at landbetweenthelakes.us.

This circumnavigation of the LBL peninsula is what I call the Land Between the Lakes Paddle Route, the best flatwater paddling area in middle America. The route begins on Kentucky Lake at Boswell Landing Lake Access in Tennessee. Paddlers then head north along Kentucky Lake, passing many big bays while heading north into Kentucky. Lake accesses and campgrounds

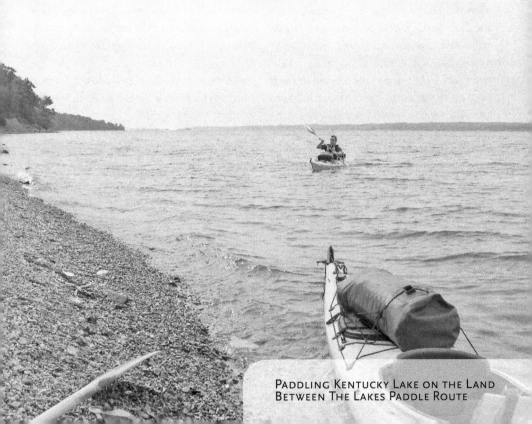

PADDLING KENTUCKY LAKE ON THE LAND
BETWEEN THE LAKES PADDLE ROUTE

occasionally break wild shoreline. The Kentucky Dam eventually comes into view. Here, paddlers take Barkley Canal, joining Kentucky Lake to Lake Barkley. Paddlers may experience a strong current here. Which way this current flows depends on which watershed—the Tennessee River or the Cumberland River—has received more rainfall recently.

Paddlers leave the canal, heading east, past Kuttawa Landing Lake Access. Beyond here, Lake Barkley turns south, and paddlers pass the largest bays of Barkley. Islands appear more frequently south of the US 68/KY 80 bridge. Finally, paddlers reenter the Volunteer State and end the paddle route at the boat launch near Gatlin Point Campground. From here, it is but 10 miles by road to Boswell Landing.

⟡ MAPS RUSHING CREEK, FENTON, FAIRDEALING, BIRMINGHAM POINT, GRAND RIVERS, EDDYVILLE, MONT, CANTON, LINTON (USGS); LAND BETWEEN THE LAKES NATIONAL RECREATION AREA MAP

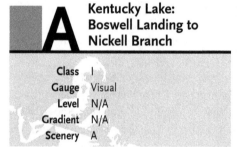

A Kentucky Lake: Boswell Landing to Nickell Branch

Class	I
Gauge	Visual
Level	N/A
Gradient	N/A
Scenery	A

69A **DESCRIPTION** The LBL Paddle Route is broken into two segments, Kentucky Lake and Lake Barkley. This first segment begins at Boswell Landing and travels north for 35 miles along the northernmost end of Kentucky Lake. Add 1 more mile passing through the Barkley Canal, the canal connecting Kentucky Lake and Lake Barkley. Boswell Landing makes for a good starting spot with its courtesy dock and boat ramp. From here, paddlers can see far north up Kentucky Lake. On entering the water, paddlers will be surprised at the width of the river—easily a mile wide. This width can cause problems if a big wind kicks up. However, the biggest surprise may be the changing character of the wild shoreline—hilly, tree-covered banks, rock bluffs, clay bluffs, and gravel bars all melded into a winding border between water and land.

There is so much shoreline to explore—deep bays with numerous arms leading up quiet coves cutting deep into the heart of LBL beg to be paddled. On the main lake, civilization is barely visible across the water. Occasional giant barge loads pushed by humming tugs ply the old bed of the Tennessee River channel. Pleasure boaters and fishing boats will be seen, especially on weekends.

Pine Bluff stands far above the lake 5 miles north of Boswell Landing. Ginger Bay Lake Access lies 2 miles north of the bluff. No services are offered. The gravel bars on the main shoreline are your best bet for camping on Kentucky Lake. The landings are easy. Enter Kentucky just beyond Rushing Creek. A large shoreline sign marks the boundary. Anglers must have a fishing license for each state in which they are fishing.

Redd Hollow Lake Access lies in a cove 2 miles north of the state line. Kentucky Lake narrows a bit. Beyond here, the Eggners Ferry Bridge becomes visible. Fenton Campground (with potable water) is on the LBL shoreline just before the bridge. Kenlake State Park is on the western shore by the bridge. The lake widens again north of the bridge. Here, deeply cut bays are interspersed along the main shoreline. Exploration opportunities are numerous along this wild shore. The rocky point just south of Higgins Bay makes for a good breaking spot.

Land Between the Lakes Paddle Route

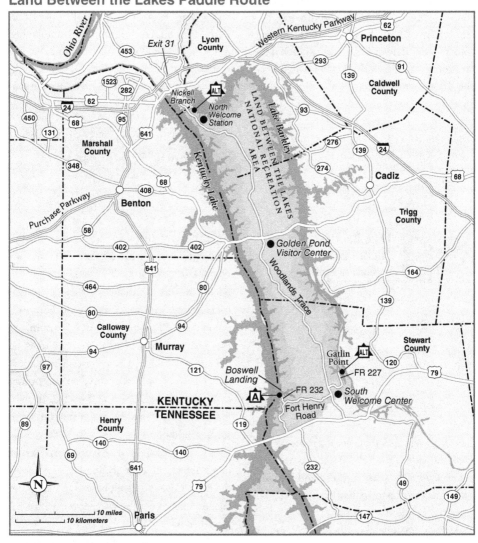

Things become more developed far north. Smith Bay, part of Birmingham Ferry campground, 28 miles north of Boswell, marks the beginning of this developed area. Just ahead is large Hillman Ferry Campground, which offers water and hot showers. The north end of the campground is closer to the main lake channel. Twin Lakes Lake Access and Moss Creek Day-Use Area come next. By now, the Kentucky Dam may be visible. Pass high bluffs then metal pillars used to hold barges just before reaching the Barkley Canal, 35 miles north of Boswell Landing. Pass through the rock-lined connector and keep along the LBL shoreline. Barkley Dam is visible to your left after passing through the canal. Ahead on your right is Nickell Branch Lake Access and the end of the Kentucky Lake section.

✧ **SHUTTLE** To reach the take out from Exit 31 on I-24 near Lake City, head south on KY 453 for 7 miles. KY 453 becomes the Trace once it enters Land Between the Lakes National Recreation Area. The North Welcome Station will be on your right. From the North Welcome Station at Land Between the Lakes, take the Trace north 1.0 mile to Forest Road 102. Turn right on FR 102 and follow it 0.9 mile to dead-end at Nickell Branch landing. To reach the put-in, backtrack to the Trace and head south on the Trace to take FR 230, Fort Henry Road. Turn right on Fort Henry Road and follow it 4.1 miles to FR 232. Turn right on FR 232 and follow it 0.1 mile to FR 233. Turn right on FR 233 and follow it 1.2 miles to dead-end at Boswell Landing.

✧ **GAUGE** This section of Kentucky Lake is floatable year-round.

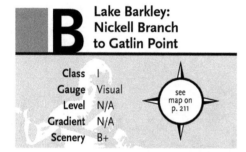

B Lake Barkley: Nickell Branch to Gatlin Point

Class	I
Gauge	Visual
Level	N/A
Gradient	N/A
Scenery	B+

see map on p. 211

69B **DESCRIPTION** The second portion of the LBL Paddle Route is longer—50 miles, and that is traveling in this shortest route possible with no side trips. Lake Barkley is narrower than Kentucky Lake. Long, slender islands break its lower part, potentially causing navigational problems. Getting around Kentucky Lake is simpler: head north and keep the LBL shoreline to your right. Barkley's shoreline is more continually forested with few gravel bars and fewer bluffs. The densely forested banks make finding a backcountry campsite more challenging. Look at the mouths of valleys entering the lake—they tend to offer more level ground. Be prepared to look around for a suitable campsite. However, the numerous lake accesses can always function as backup campsites. The old Cumberland River channel swings all over Lake Barkley. Barges and bigger boats often follow this channel because Barkley is riddled with shallows that normally do not affect self-propelled boats.

Begin this segment at Nickell Branch Lake Access and work east along the northern end of LBL. Large bays, like Demumbers Bay, characterize this area. Younger trees on the shoreline tell of a heavily settled area just now returning to forest. Curve north, coming to Kuttawa Lake Access at 8 miles. Beyond the landing, the paddle route turns south and stays southbound for the rest of the route, shortly passing Eddyville Ferry Lake Access in a hollow. Interestingly, the big building of the Kentucky State Penitentiary lies across the lake here. Look for the water tower with KSP inscribed on it.

Big bays cut into LBL below Kuttawa. A portion of Cravens Bay Campground stands on the main shoreline at 17 miles. Here you can get potable water. Ahead are the first islands. The now-closed Silo Overlook on the LBL shoreline marks the Environmental Education (EE) Area. No camping is allowed in the EE Area, which is bordered on the north by Fulton Bay and on the south bay part of Taylor Bay. Be aware that camping is allowed at Taylor Bay Lake Access at mile 23.

Paddlers may want to consider entering Crooked Creek Bay, which offers good fishing and a developed campground on the far side of Energy Lake Dam. This would require a carry over the low dam. Keeping south on the now narrower main lake, reach the US 68/KY 80 bridge at 30 miles. Devils Elbow Lake Access is just south of here. The shoreline remains wild for 4 miles below Bacon Creek Lake Access. Islands appear with regularity at this point. Smart paddlers will positively identify Neville Bay at 46 miles (you can see the grassy lake access from the main lake) and keep the LBL shoreline within view. Otherwise, you may miss the Gatlin Point Campground ramp and take-out, because several very long, narrow islands block Gatlin Point from view if paddlers follow the main river channel. The Gatlin Point boat ramp, at 85 miles, marks the end of the LBL Paddle Route.

✧ **SHUTTLE** To reach the put-in from Exit 31 on I-24 near Lake City, head south on KY 453 for 7 miles. KY 453 becomes the Trace once it enters Land Between the Lakes National Recreation Area. The North Welcome Station will be on your right. From the North Welcome Station at Land Between the Lakes, take the Trace north 1 mile to FR 102. Turn right on FR 102 and follow it 0.9 mile to dead-end at Nickell Branch landing. To reach the Gatlin Point take out from the North Welcome Station, take the Trace south to FR 227. Turn left on FR 227 and follow it 2 miles. Veer left on FR 229 and follow it 1.5 miles, and the campground will be on your left. The landing is on the far side of a low dam.

✧ **GAUGE** This section of Lake Barkley is floatable year-round.

GPS COORDINATES

ACCESS	LATITUDE	LONGITUDE
BOSWELL LANDING	N36° 31.178'	W88° 1.439
NICKELL BRANCH	N36° 59.259'	W88° 11.920'
GATLIN POINT	N36° 33.805'	W87° 54.424'

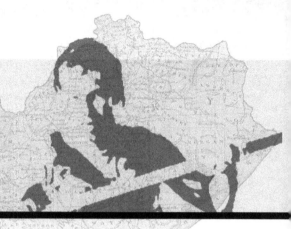

PART TEN
STREAMS OF THE JACKSON PURCHASE

70 BAYOU DU CHIEN

◇ **OVERVIEW** The Bayou du Chien is a diminutive, willow- and cypress-canopied stream that flows west out of Graves County, draining southern Hickman and northern Fulton Counties before emptying into the Mississippi River. Although artificially channeled (dredged) at one time, nature has fought back over the years to reoccupy the banks with vegetation. The result is a beautiful, almost primeval little bayou that has a generally unobstructed, navigable channel.

◇ **MAPS** WATER VALLEY, CRUTCHFIELD, CLINTON, CAYCE, HICKMAN (USGS)

KY 1283 to KY 239

Class	I
Gauge	Web
Level	Min. 100–Max. N/A (cfs)
Gradient	2.7'
Scenery	B

◇ **DESCRIPTION** Bayou du Chien runs over a mud bottom within the confines of 5-foot banks through flat farmland. At high water, the Bayou broadens from its normal 30 feet to more than a half mile in certain places, creating an immense lowland swamp and making it difficult to stay on course. At lower levels, the stream can be surprisingly clear as it winds between sandbars and around log piles. Runnable downstream of the KY 307 bridge from late fall through June, access is generally good. The level of difficulty is Class I. Dangers consist of numerous deadfalls, droves of mosquitoes, and the possibility of getting lost at higher water. The most scenic section of Bayou du Chien lies

Bayou du Chien

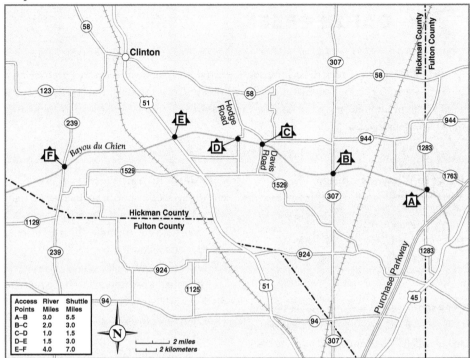

Access Points	River Miles	Shuttle Miles
A–B	3.0	5.5
B–C	2.0	3.0
C–D	1.0	1.5
D–E	1.5	3.0
E–F	4.0	7.0

between KY 307 and KY 239. In this section particularly, wildlife abounds.

◇ SHUTTLE To reach the take-out from Clinton, head south on US 51, then split right onto Washington Street. Turn right onto KY 780 and follow it 0.3 mile. Turn right onto KY 1037 and follow it 0.6 mile. Turn left onto KY 123 North and go 1.3 miles. Turn left onto KY 239 South and follow it 2.3 miles to the bridge over Bayou

du Chien. To reach the put-in from the take-out, continue on KY 239 South 0.8 mile. Turn left onto KY 1529 East and follow it 9.8 miles. Turn left onto Rose Road and travel 3.9 miles. Turn left onto KY 1283 and follow it 0.4 mile to the bridge over Bayou du Chien.

◇ GAUGE The USGS gauge is Bayou du Chien near Clinton. The minimum level should be 100 cfs.

GPS COORDINATES

ACCESS	LATITUDE	LONGITUDE	ACCESS	LATITUDE	LONGITUDE
A	N36° 36.28'	W88° 49.03'	D	N36° 37.712'	W88° 55.643'
B	N36° 36.758'	W88° 52.313'	E	N36° 37.725'	W88° 57.865'
C	N36° 37.549'	W88° 54.795'	F	N36° 36.913'	W89° 1.801'

71   OBION CREEK

◇ **OVERVIEW** Obion Creek drains the south-central portion of the Jackson Purchase area in far western Kentucky. Originating at the bottom of Graves County, the creek flows over a mud bottom into Hickman and Carlisle Counties before heading southwest to empty into the Mississippi River.

◇ **MAPS** Oakton, Wolf Island, Hickman (USGS)

US 51 to Whaynes Corner

Class	I
Gauge	Visual
Level	Min. 3.5'–Max. N/A
Gradient	2.5'
Scenery	D

◇ **DESCRIPTION** Averaging 30 feet in width, Obion Creek is a dense tangle of cypress trees and deadfalls. Recommended only to those adventurous souls who don't mind paddling in a cloud of mosquitoes or portaging every 200 feet, Obion Creek offers the utmost in flatwater paddling hardship. Banks are from 5 to 8 feet high and broaden onto wide, flat floodplains forested with oak and hickory trees. The creek itself is dense with scrub vegetation and almost completely overhung with trees—primarily willows. Obion Creek is runnable (has sufficient water) from US 51 to its mouth from November to mid-June. Access can be challenging, though the US 51 bridge (A) and KY 58 bridge (B) aren't bad. Deadfalls and flash flooding present the greatest hazards to navigation.

◇ **SHUTTLE** To reach the take-out from Clinton, head south on US 51, then split right onto Washington Street. Turn right onto KY 780 and follow it 0.3 mile. Turn right onto KY 1037 and follow it 0.6 mile. Turn left onto KY 123 North and go 2.9 miles. Stay left to join Hickman Road and follow it 3.7 miles to reach the bridge over Obion Creek, just before Hickman Road makes a sharp right. To reach the put-in from the take-out, return to Clinton and head north on US 51 for 6.5 miles to the bridge over US 51.

◇ **GAUGE** There is a gauge on the downstream side of the US 51 bridge. Minimum reading should be 3.5 feet.

GPS Coordinates

ACCESS	LATITUDE	LONGITUDE
A	N36° 45.517'	W89° 0.156'
B	N36° 43.499'	W89° 2.605'
C	N36° 40.190'	W89° 5.703'
D	N36° 38.958'	W89° 7.345'

Obion Creek

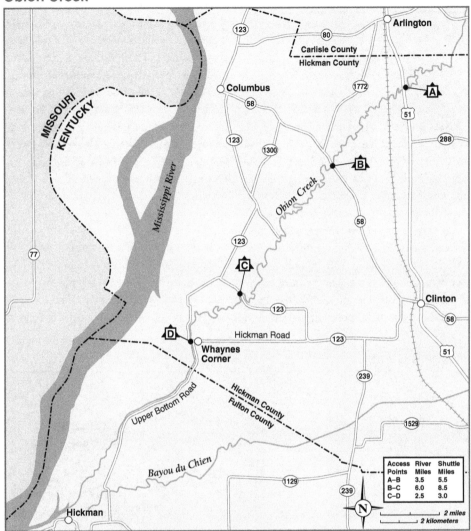

72 MAYFIELD CREEK

◇ OVERVIEW Mayfield Creek originates in Calloway County and flows northwest through Graves and McCracken Counties before becoming the Ballard–Carlisle County line and emptying into the Mississippi River south of Cairo, Illinois.

◇ MAPS WESTPLAINS, HICKORY, MELBER, LOVELACEVILLE, BLANDVILLE, WICKCLIFFE (USGS)

East of Hickory to KY 121

Class	I
Gauge	Visual
Level	Min. N/A–Max. N/A
Gradient	3.8'
Scenery	B

◇ **DESCRIPTION** Only runnable north of the city of Mayfield, the creek is distinguished by the purity of its water and the abundance of wildlife along its banks. Flowing through flat farmland, over a sand and clay bottom beneath steep 10-foot banks, Mayfield Creek is serenely enclosed by cypress, willow, and sycamore trees and by thick scrub vegetation. The level of difficulty is Class I throughout, but sandbars and the twisting nature of the stream make paddling interesting. Averaging 35–55 feet in width, the creek can be run from just east of Hickory (north of Mayfield) downstream from late fall to early summer. Access is generally good. Dangers consist of deadfalls, beaver dams, and flash flooding that turns the floodplain into a large swamp. Paddlers who may ply the Mayfield during hunting season are advised to wear bright clothing because the area is a perennial favorite of hunters. Recommended paddling sections are from east of Hickory to US 62. Numerous access points off KY 1241 make trips of varied distances easy. West of US 62, access is more difficult and the stream not nearly as pristine or beautiful.

◇ **SHUTTLE** To reach the take-out from Exit 24 on the Purchase Parkway in Mayfield, take KY 121 North 20.1 miles to the bridge over Mayfield Creek. To reach the put-in from the take-out, return to Mayfield and take US 45 from

Mayfield Creek

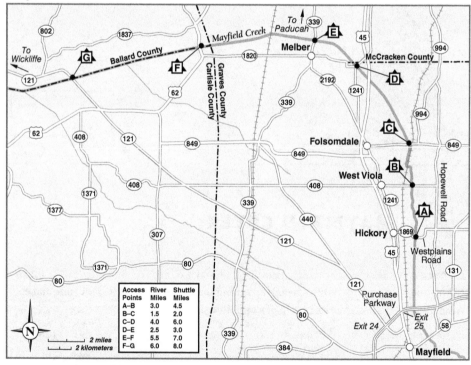

Access Points	River Miles	Shuttle Miles
A–B	3.0	4.5
B–C	1.5	2.0
C–D	4.0	6.0
D–E	2.5	3.0
E–F	5.5	7.0
F–G	6.0	8.0

Exit 25 on the Purchase Parkway. Follow US 45 North 1.8 miles. Veer right onto KY 1241 North and follow it 2.1 miles. Turn right onto Westplains Road/KY 1869 and follow it 1.1 miles to reach the bridge over Mayfield Creek.

◇ GAUGE Visual. Mayfield Creek is usually runnable from late fall through early summer.

GPS COORDINATES

ACCESS	LATITUDE	LONGITUDE	ACCESS	LATITUDE	LONGITUDE
A	N36° 49.135'	W88° 37.821'	E	N36° 57.430'	W88° 43.345'
B	N36° 51.344'	W88° 37.998'	F	N36° 57.180'	W88° 49.519'
C	N36° 53.128'	W88° 38.180'	G	N36° 55.785'	W88° 56.575'
D	N36° 56.345'	W88° 41.053'			

73 CLARKS RIVER

◇ OVERVIEW The Clarks River drains Marshall, Graves, and McCracken Counties southeast of Paducah. Except for the 3 or 4 miles near Paducah, upstream of its mouth at the Tennessee River, the Clarks River is beautiful and engaging. Wildlife abounds, particularly beaver, raccoon, deer, and (during the fall) duck.

◇ MAPS ELVA, SYMSONIA, PADUCAH EAST (USGS)

East Fork to Mouth of Clarks River

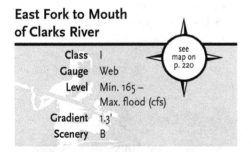

Class	I
Gauge	Web
Level	Min. 165 – Max. flood (cfs)
Gradient	1.3'
Scenery	B

see map on p. 220

◇ DESCRIPTION Running through flat farmand woodland (and through what is swamp during the rainy season), the river flows between steep mud banks crowded with cypress, sycamore, willow, maple, and scrub vegetation. The stream is exceptionally winding and continually loops back on itself. Oxbow lakes are common and are worth visiting to observe the wildlife. The Clarks River is runnable downstream of the bridge on the Sharpe-Elva Road (A) on the East Fork, to its mouth at the Tennessee River from mid-fall to early summer. The West Fork of the Clarks River is not runnable. The Clarks's average width is 35–45 feet on the East Fork and 60 feet below the confluence of the forks. The level of difficulty is Class I with deadfalls and seasonal flooding posing the major dangers. On the East Fork especially, it is very easy to get lost when the river has overflowed the adjoining floodplain. Current in the upper sections is unexpectedly swift for a low-gradient stream of western Kentucky, but it halts abruptly about 6 miles upstream of the mouth where the backwater of the Tennessee River begins, around Sheehan Bridge (C),

Clarks River

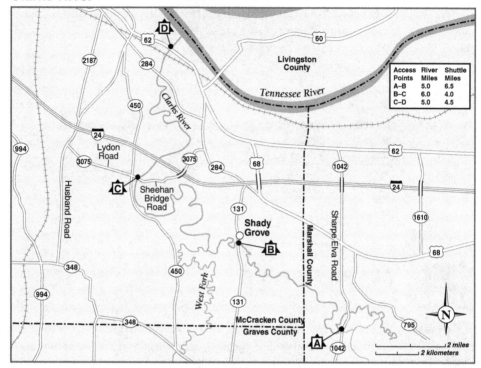

Access Points	River Miles	Shuttle Miles
A–B	5.0	6.5
B–C	6.0	4.0
C–D	5.0	4.5

where a launch has been established. In this same section, some powerboats are encountered, and the stream sacrifices much of its attractiveness as it approaches Paducah. Scrub vegetation, insects, and streamside private property limit canoe-camping possibilities. Access is good. Near Shady Grove and KY 131, check nearby Reidland Ballpark, north of the river, as attempts have been underway to create a paddler launch.

◇ **SHUTTLE** To reach the take-out from Exit 16 on I-24, just east of Paducah, take US 68 West 0.8 mile. Turn left to join US 62 West and follow it 3.3 miles to the spur road leading to the boat ramp under the US 62 bridge over Clarks Creek. To reach the put-in from the take-out, backtrack to Exit 16 and continue on US 68 East 2.7 miles. Turn right onto Sharpe Elva Road and follow it 1.9 miles to the bridge over the Clarks River.

◇ **GAUGE** The USGS gauge is Clarks River at Almo. The minimum reading should be 165 cfs.

GPS Coordinates

ACCESS	LATITUDE	LONGITUDE
A	N36° 56.423'	W88° 27.995'
B	N36° 58.307'	W88° 30.906'
C	N36° 59.769'	W88° 33.775'
D	N37° 2.617'	W88° 32.835'

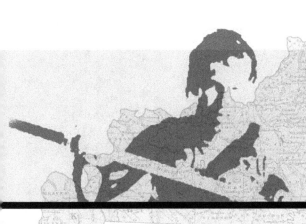

PART ELEVEN
WATERS OF SPECIAL MENTION

74 BALLARD WILDLIFE MANAGEMENT AREA

◇ **OVERVIEW** Located in Ballard County in the far northwestern corner of the state along the Ohio River, the Ballard Wildlife Management Area (BWMA) is easily one of the most unusual water resources in the state of Kentucky. Consisting of more than 15 oxbow lakes and cypress bogs, the refuge-hunting area is home to countless deer, beaver, waterfowl, songbirds, and reptiles.

◇ **MAPS** OLMSTEAD, BARLOW (USGS)

Ballard County

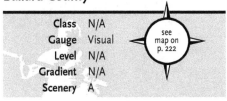

Class	N/A
Gauge	Visual
Level	N/A
Gradient	N/A
Scenery	A

see map on p. 222

◇ **DESCRIPTION** Captivating in its primeval beauty, sometimes ghostly and mysterious with imposing cypress standing guard over a watery carpet of lotus, the BWMA is always alive and always alluring. For the paddler, whose kayak or canoe allows exploring without restriction, the lakes of the BWMA offer unparalleled serenity and an opportunity to observe firsthand myriad forms of bird, animal, and fish life. Small boat ramps have been added along several of the lakes. Lakes and bogs are generally separated by only a few hundred feet, so portaging from one lake to another is not difficult. All paddling is on lakes with no moving current, and motorboat traffic is light, with BWMA regulations forbidding the use of all but silent electric motors. There are no hazards

Ballard Wildlife Management Area

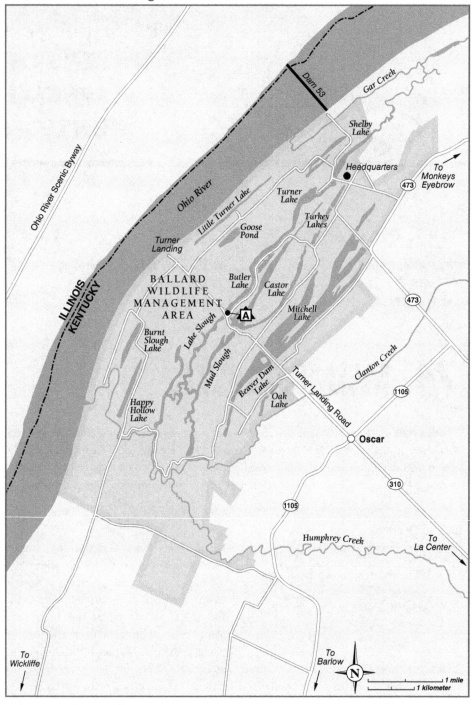

to navigation. Insects and mosquitoes represent the only potential nuisance.

⟡ SHUTTLE To reach the wildlife management area from Barlow, leave US 60 on KY 1105 and follow it north 6.5 miles. Turn left onto Turner Landing Road and enter the series of lakes with multiple accesses.

⟡ GAUGE Most lakes can be paddled all year.

GPS COORDINATES

ACCESS	LATITUDE	LONGITUDE
A	N37° 9.525'	W89° 3.348'

75 RED RIVER OF LOGAN COUNTY

⟡ OVERVIEW Kentucky has two Red Rivers. This Red River is the north fork of the Red River of Tennessee, originating in Simpson County (KY) and Robertson County (TN). This Red River flows west along the Kentucky–Tennessee border through Logan County, ultimately returning to Tennessee, emptying into the Cumberland River near Clarksville.

⟡ MAPS PRICES MILL, ADAIR, DOT, ALLENSVILLE (USGS)

Prices Mill to Tennessee State Line

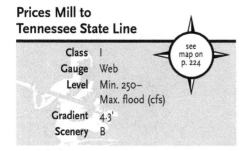

Class	I
Gauge	Web
Level	Min. 250– Max. flood (cfs)
Gradient	4.3'
Scenery	B

see map on p. 224

⟡ DESCRIPTION Runnable below Prices Mill from early November through mid-June, the Red River meanders through flat and rolling farm country and woodland and is not often paddled. The riverbed is of rock, sand, and clay with lushly vegetated banks of varying steepness. The stream is very tranquil, with a slow current and several varieties of trees (including sycamores) shading the water. Access is easy at the KY 591 bridge west of Adairville (E). Watch out for the low dam just below this access. The dam can be avoided by putting in at Logan Mill

Road (F). At the KY 591 bridge at Prices Mill (A), access is much improved over times past. Now a river access leads just off KY 591 on the north side of the river, down to the old mill dam just above the Prices Mill Bridge. Other access points include the KY 765 bridge (B) and the KY 1308 bridge (C). The US 431 bridge (D) is a tough access. The Red River averages 60–70 feet in width with occasional small islands and gravel bars dividing the river into ribbons. No obstructions other than an infrequent deadfall are in the river. It is 9 miles from Prices Mill to the KY 1308 bridge, 3 more miles to the US 431 bridge, 8 more miles to the KY 1041 bridge, and 7 more miles to the KY 102 bridge.

⟡ SHUTTLE To reach the take-out from US 431 in Adairville, take Gallatin Street/KY 591 for 5 miles to turn left on KY 96 South and follow it 6 miles. Turn left onto KY 102 South and go 2 miles, entering Tennessee to reach the bridge

Red River of Logan County

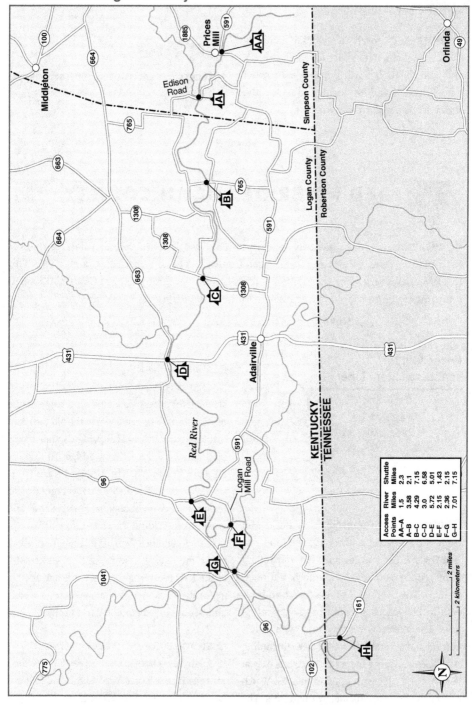

Access Points	River Miles	Shuttle Miles
AA–A	1.5	2.3
A–B	3.58	2.1
B–C	4.29	7.15
C–D	3.0	6.58
D–E	5.72	5.01
E–F	2.15	1.43
F–G	2.36	2.15
G–H	7.01	7.15

over the Red River. To reach the put-in from the take-out, backtrack to Adairville, then take KY 591 East 8.3 miles to cross the bridge over the Red River. Immediately turn right after the bridge and reach a rough access.

◆ **GAUGE** The USGS gauge is Red River at Port Royal, TN. The minimum reading should be 250 cfs for parts of the river west of Adairville and 350 cfs to run the Red east of Adairville.

GPS COORDINATES

ACCESS	LATITUDE	LONGITUDE
AA	N36° 40.932'	W86° 43.749'
A	N36° 41.422'	W86° 44.914'
B	N36° 41.253'	W86° 47.114'
C	N36° 41.312'	W86° 49.575'
D	N36° 42.066'	W86° 51.693'
E	N36° 41.560'	W86° 55.317'
F	N36° 40.698'	W86° 55.927'
G	N36° 40.593'	W86° 57.119'
H	N36° 38.430'	W86° 58.800'

76 HARRODS CREEK OF OLDHAM AND JEFFERSON COUNTIES

◆ **OVERVIEW** Harrods Creek originates in western Henry County and flows southwest through Oldham and Jefferson Counties before emptying into the Ohio River in northeastern Louisville.

◆ **MAPS** LAGRANGE, OWEN, ANCHORAGE, JEFFERSONVILLE (USGS)

KY 53 to the Ohio River

Class	I–II
Gauge	Visual
Level	Min. 180–
	Max. flood (cfs)
Gradient	11'
Scenery	B

see map on p. 226

◆ **DESCRIPTION** Harrods Creek is runnable from late November to early May downstream of KY 53 (A), and all year between the bridge at KY 329 (D) and the Ohio River (E). Harrods Creek is a pleasant Class I (II) run that winds between large boulders at the bottom of an intimate, wooded gorge. In spite of ever-encroaching Louisville, the creek, averaging 25–40 feet wide, still seems secluded and almost pristine in its rugged setting, though less so on its lower reaches near the Ohio River. Rapids never exceed an easy Class II in difficulty (and most wash out at very high water), and dangers are limited to an occasional deadfall. Access is good. After heavy rains, there is sometimes sufficient water to paddle Harrods Creek above KY 53. This is neither practicable nor safe, however, due to occasional cattle gates (fences) crossing the stream. It is 5.7 miles from the KY 53 bridge to the KY 393 bridge, 7 more miles to the KY 1694 bridge, 8.5 miles farther to the KY 329 bridge, and 8.5 miles farther to the Ohio River.

◆ **SHUTTLE** To reach the take-out from Exit 22 on I-264 northeast of Louisville, take US 42 East 2.9 miles. Turn left onto Wolf Pen Branch and follow it 0.7 mile, then make a sharp right onto River Road. Follow River Road 0.2 mile to the bridge over Harrods Creek and a marina and boat ramp on the right just after the bridge.

Harrods Creek of Oldham and Jefferson Counties

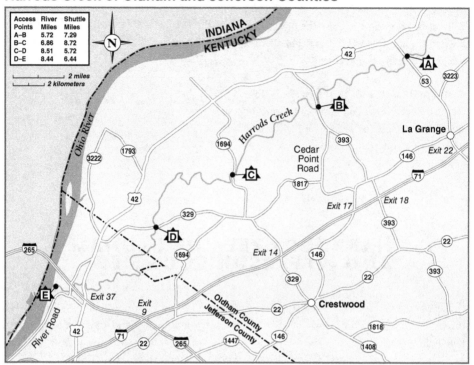

Access Points	River Miles	Shuttle Miles
A–B	5.72	7.29
B–C	6.86	8.72
C–D	8.51	5.72
D–E	8.44	6.44

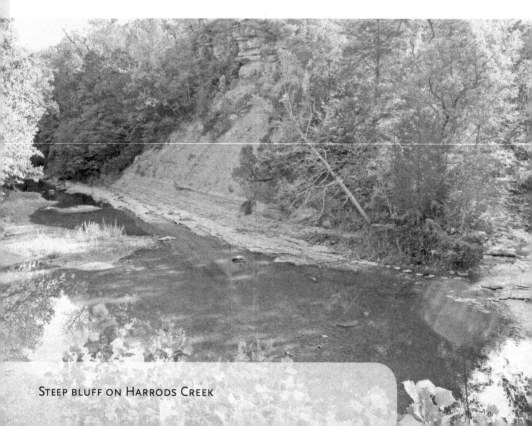

STEEP BLUFF ON HARRODS CREEK

To reach the put-in from the take-out, keep north on River Road for 1.5 miles to reach US 42. Turn left and take US 42 East for 14 miles. Turn right onto KY 53 and follow it 0.8 mile to reach the bridge over Harrods Creek.

⟡ **GAUGE** Check Harrods Creek for runnability from November to early May and after heavy rains.

GPS Coordinates

ACCESS	LATITUDE	LONGITUDE
A	N38° 26.834'	W85° 24.540'
B	N38° 25.310'	W85° 28.056'
C	N38° 23.253'	W85° 31.460'
D	N38° 21.665'	W85° 34.495'
E	N38° 19.870'	W85° 38.480'

 # 77 LITTLE KENTUCKY RIVER

⟡ **OVERVIEW** The Little Kentucky River originates in Henry County and flows northeast, draining portions of Trimble and Carroll Counties before emptying into the Ohio River near Carrollton.

⟡ **MAPS** SMITHFIELD, BEDFORD, CAMPBELLSBURG (USGS)

Sulphur to KY 316

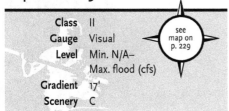

Class	II
Gauge	Visual
Level	Min. N/A– Max. flood (cfs)
Gradient	17'
Scenery	C

see map on p. 229

⟡ **DESCRIPTION** Tree lined with a rock-and-mud bottom and banks of varying steepness averaging 5 feet in height, the Little Kentucky River is runnable downstream of KY 157 (A) from mid-November to late April or early May. The most popular section, between Sulphur and US 421 (C), is a bouncy, Class II whitewater run when the water is up. Scenery is pleasant, with rolling, grazing land flanking the stream and occasional exposed rock cliffs. Dangers to paddlers include numerous deadfalls and a dam that must be portaged just above the KY 3175 bridge (B). The portage is on river right. Access is good for the section recommended.

⟡ **SHUTTLE** To reach the take-out from Exit 34 on I-71 north of Sulphur, take US 421 South 4.1 miles to the bridge over the Little Kentucky River. To reach the put-in from the take-out, backtrack on US 421 North toward the interstate, driving 3.6 miles to turn right onto KY 1606 for 3 miles. Turn right onto KY 157 and travel a short distance to the bridge over the Little Kentucky River.

⟡ **GAUGE** The river is a catch-as-catch-can proposition. Paddlers have to visually check the water before running.

GPS Coordinates

ACCESS	LATITUDE	LONGITUDE
A	N38° 29.696'	W85° 16.496'
B	N38° 32.910'	W85° 18.151
C	N38° 33.640'	W85° 16.590'

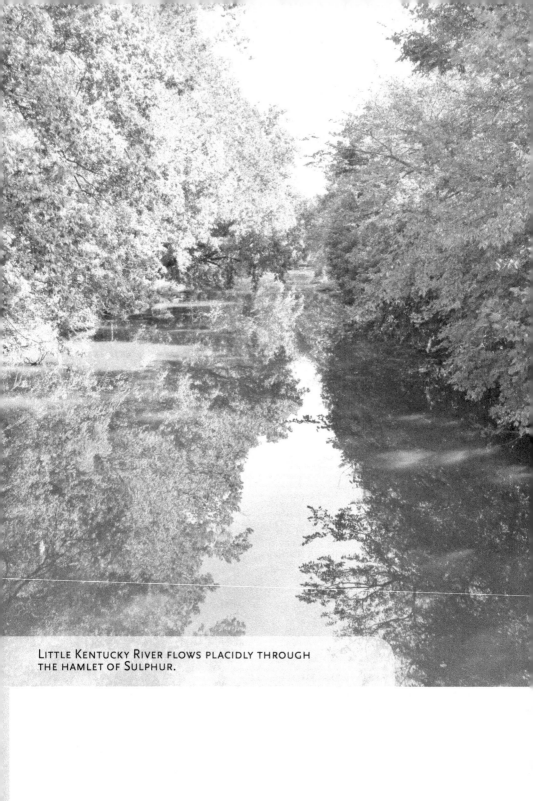

LITTLE KENTUCKY RIVER FLOWS PLACIDLY THROUGH THE HAMLET OF SULPHUR.

Little Kentucky River

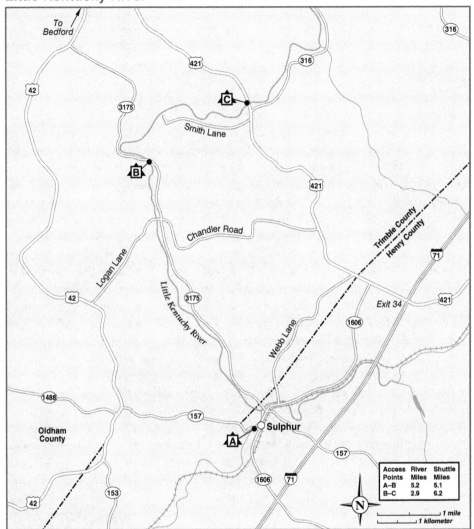

OTHER PADDLING STREAMS

◇ **OVERVIEW** In addition to the streams listed here, there are several other streams that paddling enthusiasts get on when they can. However, running these streams has been problematic—they have only been run a few times, and the runs are not well known, they rise and fall very rapidly after rains, or accesses have not been firmly established. That being said, adventurous "steep creekers" are discovering and making first descents of streams that may become standard paddling places in the future.

What follows are some creeks in transition. In the future, they may become part of the regular circuit or the topic of tales of what could be if not for lack of water, cattle fences, unfriendly landowners, and so on. Interested paddlers can check the American Whitewater Association (AWA) website (americanwhitewater.org) for the latest status on these streams. Banklick Creek, a tributary of the Licking River in Kenton County, has Class II–III water, but water quality has been a problem in the past. Cedar Branch, in Mercer County near the Shaker Village of Pleasant Hill, has Class III–IV water in a steep, walled gorge when it is up. It comes into the Kentucky River just upstream of old Lock 7. White Oak Creek, just off US 27 in Garrard County is reputed to be one of the steepest creeks run in the Bluegrass. It lies within Nature Conservancy land. The put-in is decent for the 2-mile run, but the take-out requires a 2-mile upstream paddle on the Kentucky River. White Oak Creek also holds many strainers. Glenns Creek, offering a 3-mile Class II–III run, traverses horse country near Lexington, but access is a problem. Gunpowder Creek is also a tributary of the Licking River and offers 7 miles of Class II+ water in Boone County. The beautiful creek has had water quality problems in the past. Jouett Creek, a tributary of the Kentucky River near Winchester, has an extremely small drainage—you have to practically sit in your car and watch the water to catch it at a runnable level. Rapids can be exciting and rugged because they are Class IV. Access is very limited. Roaring Paunch Creek, in the Big South Fork, has only been run a couple of times. The boulder-choked stream is very challenging, with Class IV–V+ rapids, portages, and a lot of scouting to be expected. Shawnee Run is a short creek that flows into the Kentucky River near Harrodsburg. When up, it has Class I–III (IV) rapids. One section has more than 10 cattle fences in 2 miles! Many smaller streams throughout the state offer Class I paddling in spring.

As the sport grows, adventurous canoers and kayakers will scout and run new streams, and other watercourses will undoubtedly be added to this list. If you are considering the just-mentioned streams or any other unknown waters, first check the AWA website, consult other paddlers, and assemble a team to run your creek of choice—unforeseen strainers, cattle fences, low-water bridges, and impossible rapids can turn a watery adventure into a life-or-death experience. Be a smart paddler.

OPPOSITE: THE RED RIVER OF LOGAN COUNTY
(SEE PAGE 223)

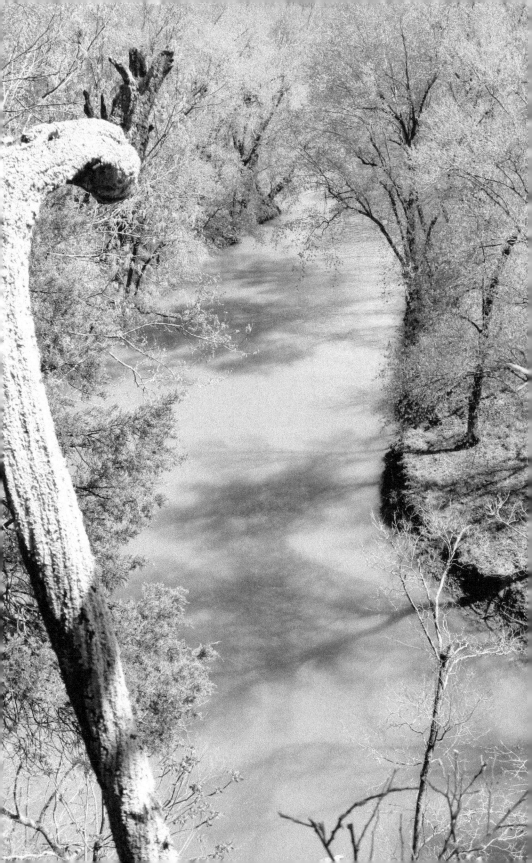

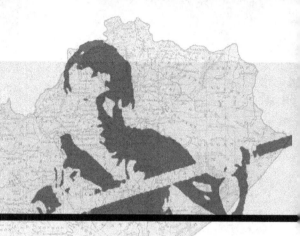

PART TWELVE
APPENDIXES

APPENDIX A:
SAFETY CODE OF AMERICAN WHITEWATER

Charlie Walbridge, *Safety Chairman* | Mark Singleton, *Executive Director*
© 1999–2016 American Whitewater, PO Box 1540, Cullowhee, NC 28723;
(866) BOAT-4-AW; info@amwhitewater.org.

INTRODUCTION

This code has been prepared using the best available information and has been reviewed by a broad cross section of whitewater experts. The code, however, is only a collection of guidelines; attempts to minimize risks should be flexible, not constrained by a rigid set of rules. Varying conditions and group goals may combine with unpredictable circumstances to require alternate procedures. This code is not intended to serve as a standard of care for commercial outfitters or guides.

I. PERSONAL PREPAREDNESS AND RESPONSIBILITY

1. Be a competent swimmer, with the ability to handle yourself underwater.

2. Wear a life jacket. A snugly fitting vest-type life preserver offers back and shoulder protection as well as the flotation needed to swim safely in whitewater.

3. Wear a solid, correctly fitted helmet when upsets are likely. This is essential in kayaks or covered canoes, and recommended for open canoeists using thigh straps and rafters running steep drops.

4. Do not boat out of control. Your skills should be sufficient to stop or reach shore before reaching danger. Do not enter a rapid unless you are reasonably sure that you can run it safely or swim it without injury.

5. Whitewater rivers contain many hazards that are not always easily recognized. The following are the most frequent killers:

    A. *High water.* The river's speed and power increase tremendously as the flow increases, raising the difficulty of most rapids. Rescue becomes progressively harder as the water rises, adding to the danger. Floating debris and strainers make even an easy rapid quite hazardous. It is often misleading to judge the river level at the put-in, since a small rise in a wide, shallow place will be multiplied many times where the river narrows. Use reliable gauge information whenever possible, and be aware that sun on snowpack, hard rain, and upstream dam releases may greatly increase the flow.

B. Cold. Cold drains your strength and robs you of the ability to make sound decisions on matters affecting your survival. Cold-water immersion, because of the initial shock and the rapid heat loss that follows, is especially dangerous. Dress appropriately for bad weather or sudden immersion in the water. When the water temperature is less than 50°F, a wetsuit or drysuit is essential for protection if you swim. Next best is wool or pile clothing under a waterproof shell. In this case, you should also carry waterproof matches and a change of clothing in a waterproof bag. If, after prolonged exposure, a person experiences uncontrollable shaking, loss of coordination, or difficulty speaking, he or she is hypothermic and needs your assistance.

C. Strainers. Brush, fallen trees, bridge pilings, undercut rocks, or anything else that allows river current to sweep through can pin boats and boaters against the obstacle. Water pressure on anything trapped this way can be overwhelming. Rescue is often extremely difficult. Pinning may occur in fast current, with little or no whitewater to warn of the danger.

D. Dams, weirs, ledges, reversals, holes, and hydraulics. When water drops over an obstacle, it curls back on itself, forming a strong upstream current that may be capable of holding a boat or swimmer. Some holes make for excellent sport; others are proven killers. Paddlers who cannot recognize the difference should avoid all but the smallest holes. Hydraulics around man-made dams must be treated with utmost respect regardless of their height or the level of the river. Despite their seemingly benign appearance, they can create an almost escape-proof trap. The swimmer's only exit from the "drowning machine" is to dive below the surface when the downstream current is flowing beneath the reversal.

E. Broaching. When a boat is pushed sideways against a rock by strong current, it may collapse and wrap. This is especially dangerous to kayak and decked-canoe paddlers; these boats will collapse, and the combination of indestructible hulls and tight outfitting may create a deadly trap. Even without entrapment, releasing pinned boats can be extremely time-consuming and dangerous. To avoid pinning, throw your weight downstream toward the rock. This allows the current to slide harmlessly underneath the hull.

6. Boating alone is discouraged. The minimum party is three people or two craft.

7. Have a frank knowledge of your boating ability, and don't attempt rivers or rapids that lie beyond that ability.

8. Be in good physical and mental condition, consistent with the difficulties that may be expected. Make adjustments for loss of skills due to age, health, fitness. Any health limitations must be explained to your fellow paddlers prior to starting the trip.

9. Be practiced in self-rescue, including escape from an overturned craft. The Eskimo roll is strongly recommended for decked boaters who run rapids Class IV or greater, or who paddle in cold environmental conditions.

10. Be trained in rescue skills, CPR, and first aid, with special emphasis on the recognizing and treating hypothermia. It may save your friend's life.

11. Carry equipment needed for unexpected emergencies, including footwear that will protect your feet when walking out, a throw rope, knife, whistle, and waterproof matches. If you wear eyeglasses, tie them on and carry a spare pair on long trips. Bring cloth repair tape on short runs and a full repair kit on isolated rivers. Do not wear bulky jackets, ponchos, heavy boots, or anything else that could reduce your ability to survive a swim.

12. Despite the mutually supportive group structure described in this code, individual paddlers are ultimately responsible for their own safety and must assume sole responsibility for the following decisions:

    A. *The decision to participate on any trip.* This includes an evaluation of the expected difficulty of the rapids under the conditions existing at the time of the put-in.

    B. *The selection of appropriate equipment,* including a boat design suited to their skills and the appropriate rescue and survival gear.

    C. *The decision to scout any rapid, and to run or portage according to their best judgment.* Other members of the group may offer advice, but paddlers should resist pressure from anyone to paddle beyond their skills. It is also their responsibility to decide whether to pass up any walk-out or take-out opportunity.

    D. *All trip participants should consistently evaluate their own and their group's safety,* voicing their concerns when appropriate and following what they believe to be the best course of action. Paddlers are encouraged to speak with anyone whose actions on the water are dangerous, whether they are a part of your group or not.

II. BOAT AND EQUIPMENT PREPAREDNESS

1. Test new and different equipment under familiar conditions before relying on it for difficult runs. This is especially true when adopting a new boat design or outfitting system. Low-volume craft may present additional hazards to inexperienced or poorly conditioned paddlers.

2. Be sure your boat and gear are in good repair before starting a trip. The more isolated and difficult the run, the more rigorous this inspection should be.

3. Install flotation bags in noninflatable craft, securely fixed in each end and designed to displace as much water as possible. Inflatable boats should have multiple air chambers and be test-inflated before launching.

4. Have strong, properly sized paddles or oars for controlling your craft. Carry sufficient spares for the length and difficulty of the trip.

5. Outfit your boat safely. The ability to exit your boat quickly is an essential component of safety in rapids. It is your responsibility to see that there is absolutely nothing to cause entrapment when coming free of an upset craft, such as the following:

    A. *Spray covers that won't release reliably* or that release prematurely.

    B. *Boat outfitting too tight to allow a fast exit,* especially in low-volume kayaks or decked canoes. This includes low-hung thwarts in canoes lacking adequate clearance for your feet and kayak footbraces which fail or allow your feet to become wedged under them.

    C. *Inadequately supported decks* that collapse on a paddler's legs when a decked boat is pinned by water pressure. Inadequate clearance with the deck because of your size or build.

D. *Loose ropes that cause entanglement.* Beware of any length of loose line attached to a whitewater boat. All items must be tied tightly and excess line eliminated; painters, throw lines, and safety-rope systems must be completely and effectively stored. Do not knot the end of a rope, as it can get caught in cracks between rocks.

6. Provide ropes that permit you to hold on to your craft so that it may be rescued. The following methods are recommended:

   A. *Kayaks and covered canoes* should have grab loops of 0.25-inch-plus rope or equivalent webbing sized to admit a normal-size hand. Stern painters are permissible if properly secured.

   B. *Open canoes* should have securely anchored bow and stern painters consisting of 8–10 feet of 0.25-inch-plus line. These must be secured in such a way that they are readily accessible but cannot come loose accidentally. Grab loops are acceptable but are more difficult to reach after an upset.

   C. *Rafts and dories* may have taut perimeter lines threaded through the loops provided. Footholds should be designed so that a paddler's feet cannot be forced through them, causing entrapment. Flip lines should be carefully and reliably stowed.

7. Know your craft's carrying capacity and how added loads affect boat handling in whitewater. Most rafts have a minimum crew size that can be added to on day trips or in easy rapids. Carrying more than two paddlers in an open canoe when running rapids is not recommended.

8. Car-top racks must be strong and attach positively to the vehicle. Lash your boat to each crossbar, then tie the ends of the boats directly to the bumpers for added security. This arrangement should survive all but the most violent vehicle accident.

III. GROUP PREPAREDNESS AND RESPONSIBILITY

1. **ORGANIZATION.** A river trip should be regarded as a common adventure by all participants, except on instructional or commercially guided trips as defined below. Participants share the responsibility for the conduct of the trip, and each participant is individually responsible for judging his or her own capabilities and for his or her own safety as the trip progresses. Participants are encouraged (but are not obligated) to offer advice and guidance for the independent consideration and judgment of others.

2. **RIVER CONDITIONS.** The group should have a reasonable knowledge of the difficulty of the run. Participants should evaluate this information and adjust their plans accordingly. Maps and guidebooks, if available, should be examined if the run is exploratory or no one is familiar with the river. The group should secure accurate flow information; the more difficult the run, the more important this will be. Be aware of possible changes in river level and how this will affect the difficulty of the run. If the trip involves tidal stretches, secure appropriate information on tides.

3. **GROUP EQUIPMENT SHOULD BE SUITED TO THE DIFFICULTY OF THE RIVER.** The group should always have a throw line available, and one line per boat is recommended on difficult runs. The list may include: carabiners, prussic loops, first aid kit, flashlight, folding saw, fire starter, guidebooks, maps, food, extra clothing, and any other rescue or survival items suggested by conditions. Each item is not required on every run, and this list is not meant to be a substitute for good judgment.

4. KEEP THE GROUP COMPACT, BUT MAINTAIN SUFFICIENT SPACING TO AVOID COLLISIONS. If the group is large, consider dividing into smaller groups or using the "buddy system" as an additional safeguard. Space yourselves closely enough to permit good communication, but not so close as to interfere with one another in rapids.

A. *A point paddler sets the pace.* When in front, do not get in over your head. Never run drops when you cannot see a clear route to the bottom or, for advanced paddlers, a sure route to the next eddy. When in doubt, stop and scout.

B. *Keep track of all group members.* Each boat keeps the one behind it in sight, stopping if necessary. Know how many people are in your group, and take head counts regularly. No one should paddle ahead or walk out without first informing the group. Paddlers requiring additional support should stay at the center of a group and not allow themselves to lag behind in the more difficult rapids. If the group is large and contains a wide range of abilities, a "sweep boat" may be designated to bring up the rear.

C. *Courtesy.* On heavily used rivers, do not cut in front of a boater running a drop. Always look upstream before leaving eddies to run or play. Never enter a crowded drop or eddy when no room for you exists. Passing other groups in a rapid may be hazardous: it's often safer to wait upstream until the group ahead has passed.

5. FLOAT PLAN. If the trip is into a wilderness area or for an extended period, plans should be filed with a responsible person who will contact the authorities if you are overdue. It may be wise to establish checkpoints along the way where civilization could be contacted if necessary. Knowing the location of possible help and preplanning escape routes can speed rescue.

6. DRUGS. The use of alcohol or mind-altering drugs before or during river trips is not recommended. These substances dull reflexes, reduce decision-making ability, and may interfere with important survival reflexes.

7. INSTRUCTIONAL OR COMMERCIALLY GUIDED TRIPS. In contrast to the common adventure-trip format, these trip formats involve a boating instructor or commercial guide who assumes some of the responsibilities normally exercised by the group as a whole, as appropriate under the circumstances. These formats recognize that instructional or commercially guided trips may involve participants who lack significant experience in whitewater. However, as a participant acquires experience, he or she takes on increasing responsibility for his or her own safety, in accordance with what he or she knows or should know as a result of that increased experience. Also, as in all trip formats, every participant must realize and assume the risks associated with the serious hazards of whitewater rivers. It is advisable for instructors and commercial guides or their employers to acquire trip or personal liability insurance:

A. An *"instructional trip"* is characterized by a clear teacher–pupil relationship, where the primary purpose of the trip is to teach boating skills, and which is conducted for a fee.

B. A *"commercially guided trip"* is characterized by a licensed, professional guide conducting trips for a fee.

IV. GUIDELINES FOR RIVER RESCUE

1. Recover from an upset with an Eskimo roll whenever possible. Evacuate your boat immediately if there is imminent danger of being trapped against rocks, brush, or any other kind of strainer.

2. If you swim, hold on to your boat. It has much flotation and is easy for rescuers to spot. Get to the upstream end so that you cannot be crushed between a rock and your boat by the force of the current. Persons with good balance may be able to climb on top of a swamped kayak or flipped raft and paddle to shore.

3. Release your craft if this will improve your chances, especially if the water is cold or dangerous rapids lie ahead. Actively attempt self-rescue whenever possible by swimming for safety. Be prepared to assist others who may come to your aid.

    A. *When swimming in shallow or obstructed rapids, lie on your back with feet held high and pointed downstream.* Do not attempt to stand in fast-moving water; if your foot wedges on the bottom, fast water will push you under and keep you there. Get to slow or very shallow water before attempting to stand or walk. Look ahead! Avoid possible pinning situations, including undercut rocks, strainers, downed trees, holes, and other dangers, by swimming away from them.

    B. *If the rapids are deep and powerful, roll over onto your stomach and swim aggressively for shore.* Watch for eddies and slackwater, and use them to get out of the current. Strong swimmers can effect a powerful upstream ferry and get to shore fast. If the shores are obstructed with strainers or undercut rocks, however, it is safer to "ride the rapid out" until a safer escape can be found.

4. If others spill and swim, go after the boaters first. Rescue boats and equipment only if this can be done safely. While participants are encouraged (but not obligated) to assist one another to the best of their ability, they should do so only if they can, in their judgment, do so safely. The first duty of a rescuer is not to compound the problem by becoming another victim.

5. The use of rescue lines requires training; uninformed use may cause injury. Never tie yourself into either end of a line without a reliable quick-release system. Have a knife handy to deal with unexpected entanglement. Learn to place set lines effectively, to throw accurately, to belay effectively, and to properly handle a rope thrown to you.

6. When reviving a drowning victim, be aware that cold water may greatly extend survival time under water. Victims of hypothermia may have depressed vital signs, causing them to look and feel dead. Don't give up; continue CPR for as long as possible without compromising safety.

V. UNIVERSAL RIVER SIGNALS

These signals may be substituted with an alternate set of signals agreed upon by the group.

STOP: *Potential hazard ahead.* Wait for "all clear" signal before proceeding, or scout ahead. Form a horizontal bar with your outstretched arms. Those seeing the signal should pass it back to others in the party.

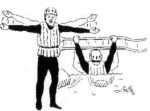

STOP: *Potential hazard ahead.*

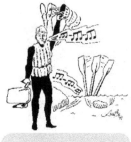

HELP: *Emergency.* Assist the signaler as quickly as possible. Give three long blasts on a police whistle while waving a paddle, helmet, or life vest over your head. If a whistle is not available, use the visual signal alone. A whistle is best carried on a lanyard attached to your life vest.

ALL CLEAR: *Come ahead.* In the absence of other directions, proceed down the center. Form a vertical bar with your paddle or one arm held high above your head (see left). Paddle blade should be turned flat for maximum visibility. To signal direction or a preferred course through a rapid around obstruction, lower the previously vertical "all clear" by 45 degrees toward the side of the river with the preferred route (see right). Never point toward the obstacle you wish to avoid.

HELP: *Emergency.*

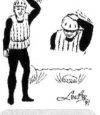

I'M OK: *I'm not hurt.*

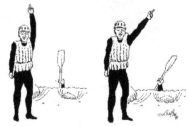

ALL CLEAR: *Come ahead.*

I'M OK: *I'm not hurt.* While holding an elbow outward toward your side, repeatedly pat the top of your head.

VI. INTERNATIONAL SCALE OF RIVER DIFFICULTY

This is the American version of a rating system used to compare river difficulty throughout the world. This system is not exact: rivers do not always fit easily into one category, and regional or individual interpretations may cause misunderstandings. It is no substitute for a guidebook or accurate first-hand descriptions of a run.

Paddlers attempting difficult runs in unfamiliar areas should act cautiously until they get a feel for the way the scale is interpreted locally. River difficulty may change each year due to fluctuations in water level, downed trees, recent floods, geological disturbances, or bad weather. Stay alert for unexpected problems!

As river difficulty increases, the danger to swimming paddlers becomes more severe. As rapids become longer and more continuous, the challenge increases. There is a difference between running an occasional Class IV rapid and dealing with an entire river of this category. Allow an extra margin of safety between skills and river ratings when the water is cold or if the river itself is remote and inaccessible.

Examples of commonly run rapids that fit each of the classifications are presented in the document "International Scale of River Difficulty: Standard Rated Rapids." This document is available online at tinyurl.com/awriverdifficultyscale. Rapids of a difficulty similar to a rapid on this list are rated the same. Rivers are also rated using this scale. A river rating should take into account many factors including the difficulty of individual rapids, remoteness, hazards, etc.

The Six Difficulty Classes:

CLASS I: *Easy.* Fast-moving water with riffles and small waves. Few obstructions, all obvious and easily missed with little training. Risk to swimmers is slight; self-rescue is easy.

CLASS II: *Novice.* Straightforward rapids with wide, clear channels that are evident without scouting. Occasional maneuvering may be required, but rocks and medium-size waves are easily missed by trained paddlers. Swimmers are seldom injured, and group assistance, while helpful, is seldom needed. Rapids that are at the upper end of this difficulty range are designated "Class II+."

CLASS III: *Intermediate.* Rapids with moderate, irregular waves that may be difficult to avoid and can swamp an open canoe. Complex maneuvers in fast current and good boat control in tight passages or around ledges are often required; large waves or strainers may be present but are easily avoided. Strong eddies and powerful current effects can be found, particularly on large-volume rivers. Scouting is advisable for inexperienced parties. Injuries while swimming are rare; self-rescue is usually easy, but group assistance may be required to avoid long swims. Rapids that are at the lower or upper end of this difficulty range are designated "Class III–" or "Class III+," respectively.

CLASS IV: *Advanced.* Intense, powerful, but predictable rapids requiring precise boat handling in turbulent water. Depending on the character of the river, it may feature large, unavoidable waves and holes or constricted passages demanding fast maneuvers under pressure. A fast, reliable eddy turn may be needed to initiate maneuvers, scout rapids, or rest. Rapids may require "must" moves above dangerous hazards. Scouting may be necessary the first time down. Risk of injury to swimmers is moderate to high, and water conditions may make self-rescue difficult. Group assistance for rescue is often essential but requires practiced skills. A strong Eskimo roll is highly recommended. Rapids that are at the upper end of this difficulty range are designated "Class IV–" or "Class IV+," respectively.

CLASS V: *Expert.* Extremely long, obstructed, or very violent rapids that expose a paddler to added risk. Drops may contain large, unavoidable waves and holes or steep, congested chutes with complex, demanding routes. Rapids may continue for long distances between pools, demanding a high level of fitness. What eddies exist may be small, turbulent, or difficult to reach. At the high end of the scale, several of these factors may be combined. Scouting is recommended but may be difficult. Swims are dangerous, and rescue is often difficult even for experts. A very reliable Eskimo roll, proper equipment, extensive experience, and practiced rescue skills are essential. Because of the large range of difficulty that exists beyond Class IV, Class 5 is an open-ended, multiple-level scale designated by 5.0, 5.1, 5.2, etc. Each of these levels is an order of magnitude more difficult than the last. Example: increasing difficulty from Class 5.0 to Class 5.1 is a similar order of magnitude as increasing from Class IV to Class 5.0.

CLASS VI: *Extreme and exploratory.* These runs have almost never been attempted and often exemplify extremes of difficulty, unpredictability, and danger. The consequences of errors are very severe, and rescue may be impossible. For teams of experts only, at favorable water levels, after close personal inspection and taking all precautions. After a Class VI rapids has been run many times, its rating may be changed to an appropriate Class 5.x rating.

APPENDIX B: RATING THE PADDLER

Bob Sehlinger, coauthor of this book, has refined and developed the paddler rating system based on previous models. Admittedly the refined system is more complex and exhaustive, but not more so than warranted by the situation.

INSTRUCTIONS: All items, except the first, carry points that may be added to obtain an overall rating. All items except "Rolling Ability" apply to both open and decked boats. Rate open and decked boat skills separately.

1. PREREQUISITE SKILLS. Before paddling on moving current, the paddler should:
- a. Have some swimming ability.
- b. Be able to paddle instinctively on nonmoving water (lake). This presumes knowledge of basic strokes.
- c. Be able to guide and control the canoe from either side without changing paddling sides.
- d. Be able to guide and control the canoe (or kayak) while paddling backwards.
- e. Be able to move the canoe (or kayak) laterally.
- f. Understand the limitations of the boat.
- g. Be practiced in "wet exit" if in a decked boat.

2. EQUIPMENT. Award points on the suitability of your equipment to whitewater. Whether you own, borrow, or rent the equipment makes no difference. Do not award points for both open canoe and decked boat.

OPEN CANOE

0 Points: Any canoe less than 15 feet for tandem; any canoe less than 14 feet for solo.

1 Point: Canoe with moderate rocker, full depth, and recurved bow; should be ≥ 15 feet in length for tandem and ≥ 14 feet in length for solo and have bow and stern painters.

2 Points: Whitewater canoe. Strong rocker design, full bow with recurve, full depth amidships, no keel; meets or exceeds minimum length requirements as described under "1 Point"; made of hand-laid fiberglass, Kevlar, Marlex, or ABS Royalex; has bow and stern painters. Canoe as described under "1 Point" but with extra flotation.

3 Points: Canoe as described under "2 Points" but with extra flotation.

DECKED BOAT, I.E. KAYAK

0 Points: Any decked boat lacking full flotation, spray skirt, or foot braces.

1 Point: Any fully equipped, decked boat with a wooden frame.

2 Points: Decked boat with full flotation, spray skirt, and foot braces; has grab loops; made of any modern composite material.

3 Points: Decked boat with foam wall reinforcement and split flotation; Neoprene spray skirt; boat has knee braces, foot braces, and grab loops.

3. EXPERIENCE. Compute the following to determine preliminary points, and then convert the preliminary points to final points according to the conversion table.

NUMBER OF DAYS SPENT EACH YEAR PADDLING:		CONVERSION TABLE	
		Preliminary Points	Final Points
Class I rivers	x 1 _____	0–20	0
Class II rivers	x 2 _____	21–60	1
Class III rivers	x 3 _____	61–100	2
Class IV rivers	x 4 _____	101–200	3
Class V rivers	x 5 _____	201–300	4
Preliminary Subtotal _____		301–up	5
+ number of years paddling experience _____			
Total Preliminary Points _____			

Note: This is the only evaluation item where it is possible to accrue more than 3 points.

4. SWIMMING
0 Points: Cannot swim.
1 Point: Weak swimmer.
2 Points: Average swimmer.
3 Points: Strong swimmer (competition level or skin diver).

5. STAMINA
0 Points: Cannot run mile in less than 10 minutes.
1 Point: Can run a mile in 7 to 10 minutes.
2 Points: Can run a mile in less than 7 minutes.

6. UPPER BODY STRENGTH
0 Points: Cannot do 15 push-ups.
1 Point: Can do 16 to 25 push-ups.
2 Points: Can do more than 25 push-ups.

7. BOAT CONTROL
0 Points: Can keep boat fairly straight.
1 Point: Can maneuver in moving water; can avoid big obstacles.
2 Points: Can maneuver in heavy water; knows how to work with the current.
3 Points: Finesse in boat placement in all types of water; uses current to maximum advantage.

8. AGGRESSIVENESS
0 Points: Does not play or work river at all.
1 Point: Timid; plays a little on familiar streams.
2 Points: Plays a lot; works most rivers hard.
3 Points: Plays in heavy water with grace and confidence.

9. EDDY TURNS
0 Points: Has difficulty making eddy turns from moderate current.
1 Point: Can make eddy turns in either direction from moderate current; can enter moderate current from eddy.
2 Points: Can catch medium eddies in either direction from heavy current; can enter very swift current from eddy.
3 Points: Can catch small eddies in heavy current.

10. FERRYING
0 Points: Cannot ferry.
1 Point: Can ferry upstream and downstream in moderate current.
2 Points: Can ferry upstream in heavy current; can ferry downstream in moderate current.
3 Points: Can ferry upstream and downstream in heavy current.

11. WATER READING
0 Points: Often in error.
1 Point: Can plan route in short rapid with several well-spaced obstacles.
2 Points: Can confidently run lead through continuous Class II; can predict the effects of waves and holes on boat.
3 Points: Can confidently run lead in continuous Class III; has knowledge to predict and handle the effects of reversals, side currents, and turning drops.

12. JUDGMENT
0 Points: Often in error.
1 Point: Has average ability to analyze difficulty of rapids.
2 Points: Has good ability to analyze difficulty of rapids and make independent judgments as to which should not be run.
3 Points: Has the ability to assist fellow paddlers in evaluating the difficulty of rapids; can explain subtleties to paddlers with less experience.

13. BRACING
0 Points: Has difficulty bracing in Class II water.
1 Point: Can correctly execute bracing strokes in Class II water.
2 Points: Can correctly brace in intermittent whitewater with medium waves and vertical drops of 3 feet or less.
3 Points: Can brace effectively in continuous whitewater with large waves and large vertical drops (4 feet and up).

14. RESCUE ABILITY
0 Points: Self-rescue in flatwater.
1 Point: Self-rescue in mild whitewater.
2 Points: Self-rescue in Class III: can assist others in mild whitewater.
3 Points: Can assist others in heavy whitewater.

15. ROLLING ABILITY
0 Points: Can only roll in pool.
1 Point: Can roll 3 out of 4 times in moving current.
2 Points: Can roll 3 out of 4 times in Class II whitewater.
3 Points: Can roll 4 out of 5 times in Class III and IV whitewater.

APPENDIX C: OUTFITTERS

BIG BUFFALO CROSSING CANOE & KAYAK

100 River Road, PO Box 985
Munfordville, KY 42765
270-774-7883; bigbuffalocrossing.com
❖ Operates on the Green River near Munfordville but also does trips through Mammoth Cave National Park.

CANOE KENTUCKY

7323 Peaks Mill Road
Frankfort, KY 40601
800-K-CANOE-I; canoeky.com
❖ Operates primarily on the Elkhorn River system but also has trips on the Green and will do special trips all over the state.

CAVE COUNTRY CANOE

856 Old Mammoth Cave Road
Cave City, KY 42127
270-773-5552; cavecountrycanoeky.com
❖ Offers a variety of trips on the Green and Nolin Rivers.

GREEN RIVER CANOEING

1145 Main St.
Brownsville, KY 42210
270-597-2031; mammothcavecanoe.com
❖ They operate on the Green River between Munfordville and Houchins Ferry, including the Green through Mammoth Cave National Park. They also run trips on the Nolin from below Nolin River Lake to the Green. Their trips last from 2 hours to 2 days.

GREEN RIVER CANOES

209 Southside Drive
Campbellsville, KY
270-789-2956
❖ Serves the Green River from below Green Lake to Munfordville. Their featured trip is the Roachville Run. Call ahead for service. They also handle custom group trips.

KENTUCKY KAYAK KOUNTRY

2040 J. H. O'Bryan Drive
Grand Rivers, KY 42045
270-362-0087
❖ This outfit, open April–October, offers guided and unguided kayak trips along the Little River, the Muddy Fork Little River, and the bays of Land Between the Lakes.

MAMMOTH CAVE CANOE & KAYAK

1240 Old Mammoth Cave Road
Cave City, KY 42127; 877-592-2663
❖ Licensed to operate in Mammoth Cave National Park, they offer canoe trips on the Green River lasting from 3 hours to 3 days.

RED RIVER ADVENTURE

606-663-5258; redriveradventure.net
❖ This outfit rents kayaks and canoes, provides shuttles for both paddlers and hikers in the Red River Gorge.

RED RIVER OUTDOORS

415 Natural Bridge Road
Slade, KY 40376
606-663-9701; redriveroutdoors.com
❖ Centered on the Red River Gorge, they offer paddling trips on various parts of the Red, rock climbing, and shuttle services for paddlers and backpackers.

ROCKCASTLE ADVENTURES CANOE LIVERY

Box 662
London, KY 40441
606-864-9407
❖ Rents canoes and offers shuttle service on Rockcastle and other local lakes and rivers.

SHELTOWEE TRACE OUTFITTERS

PO Box 1060
Whitley City, KY 42653
800-541-RAFT; ky-rafting.com
◇ Located near Cumberland Falls State Park, this group offers canoes, kayaks, and rafts, along with guided and unguided trips on the Big South Fork, Cumberland River, and Russell Fork.

THAXTON'S CANOE AND PADDLER'S INN

33 Hornbeck Road, Suite 3
Butler, KY 41006
859-472-2000; gopaddling.com
◇ Jim Thaxton and company offer day and overnight trips on the Licking River, as well as overnight trips on the South Fork Licking River.

THREE TREES CANOE AND KAYAK

300 Athens-Boonesboro Road
Winchester, KY
859-749-3227; threetreeskayak.com
◇ Located a mile from Fort Boonesborough State Park, they offer canoe and kayak trips on the historic Kentucky River.

TRADEWATER CANOE AND KAYAK

114 Lakeview Drive
Dawson Springs, KY 42408
270-871-9475
◇ Open weekends, they offer canoe and kayak rentals and shuttles on the Tradewater River.

APPENDIX D: CLUBS

KENTUCKY CLUBS

BLUEGRASS WILDWATER ASSOCIATION

PO Box 4231
Lexington, KY 40504
bluegrasswildwater.org

VIKING CANOE CLUB

Louisville, KY
vikingcanoeclub.info

NATIONAL CLUBS

AMERICAN CANOE ASSOCIATION

americancanoe.org

AMERICAN WHITEWATER ASSOCIATION

americanwhitewater.org

APPENDIX E: GLOSSARY

Back band (back rest): Provides support for the lower back while kayaking and helps with erect posture in the boat. Located behind the seat and usually made of padded fabric, plastic, or foam.

Blade: The broad part at the ends of the paddle.

Bow: The forward end of the boat.

Bulkhead: A cross-sectional wall inside a kayak, made of composite, plastic, or foam. Bulkheads provide structural support and, if sealed around the inside of the hull, can create watertight compartments for buoyancy and storage. They are sometimes also used as foot braces.

Cockpit: The enclosed central compartment on a kayak, in which the paddler sits.

Deck: The top part of a kayak that keeps the hull from filling with water.

Flotation: Waterproof compartments, foam blocks, or inflatable airbags. Flotation will help a swamped boat stay on the surface, making rescue and reentry easier.

Foot pegs (foot braces): Usually adjustable structures inside the cockpit on which a kayaker places the balls of his feet. See Bulkhead.

Hull: The structural body of the boat, the shape of which determines how the boat will perform in various conditions.

PFD: Personal flotation device. Cushions, floats, and, most importantly for kayakers, lifejackets. PFDs used in the United States must be approved by the U.S. Coast Guard and must be worn to be effective. The Coast Guard recognizes five classes of PFDs. The ACA recommends kayakers use Class III PFDs in most situations.

Rocker: The amount of curvature of a line down the middle of a kayak's hull, from bow to stern. More rocker (more curvature) usually makes a kayak more maneuverable. Less rocker tends to help the kayak track in a straight line.

Roll: The technique of righting a capsized kayak with the paddler remaining in the paddling position.

Shaft: The long, skinny part of a kayak paddle.

Sit-on-top: Kayaks without a cockpit, sit-on-tops are usually self-bailing with various seat and foot-brace configurations. Many are for recreational use, but some are designed for touring and racing.

Spray skirt (spray deck): A neoprene or nylon skirt worn by a kayaker that attaches to the rim of the cockpit. It keeps water out of the kayak.

Stern: The rear end of the kayak.

Swamp: To fill (a kayak) with water.

Thigh braces (knee braces): Usually found in whitewater and touring kayaks, these structures inside the cockpit give the paddler points of contact important for boat control.

Trim: The bow-to-stern leveling of a kayak that affects boat control. In most cases, it should be nearly level, or with the stern slightly lower in the water.

Wet exit: Coming out of a capsized kayak.

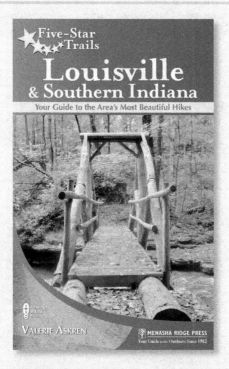

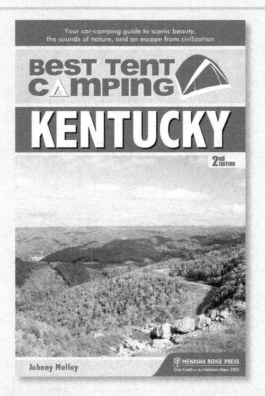

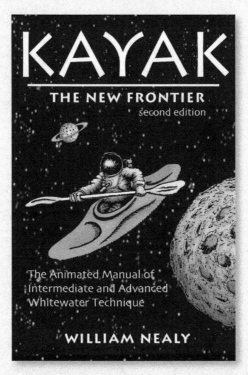

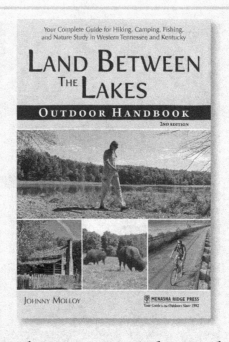

ABOUT THE AUTHORS

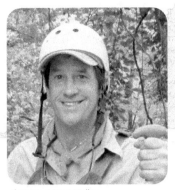

photo: Keri Anne Molloy

JOHNNY MOLLOY is an outdoor writer based in Tennessee. A native Tennessean, he was born in Memphis and moved to Knoxville in 1980 to attend the University of Tennessee. In Knoxville, he developed his love of the natural world that has since become the primary focus of his life.

It all started on a backpacking foray into the Great Smoky Mountains National Park. That first trip, though a disaster, unleashed an innate love of the outdoors that has led to his spending more than 150 nights in the wild per year over the past 30 years, backpacking and canoe camping throughout our country and abroad. In 1987, after graduating from the University of Tennessee with a degree in economics, he continued to spend ever-increasing amounts of time in the natural places, becoming more skilled in a variety of environments. Friends enjoyed his adventure stories, and one even suggested he write a book. Soon he parlayed his love of the outdoors into an occupation.

The results of his efforts are more than 60 books, ranging from hiking guides to paddling guides to camping guides to true outdoor adventure stories. His books primarily cover the Southeast but range to Colorado and Wisconsin. He has written several Kentucky guidebooks, including *Best Tent Camping: Kentucky* and *Land Between the Lakes Outdoor Handbook,* in addition to this guidebook. In recognition of his efforts at promoting Kentucky outdoors, Johnny has been named an honorary Kentucky Colonel as bestowed by Governor Steven L. Beshear.

Molloy has also written numerous magazine articles for magazines and websites, as well as newspapers. He continues to write to this day and travels extensively to all four corners of the United States, endeavoring in a variety of outdoor pursuits.

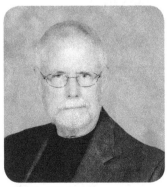

photo: Scott McGrew

BOB SEHLINGER, author of seven paddling guides and dozens of travel books, is the former president of the Eastern Professional River Outfitters Association. He also served as program director for the SAGE Inc. school of the outdoors. A native of the southeastern states, Bob has led canoeing trips throughout eastern North America from the rivers of northern Ontario, Canada, to the bayous of Louisiana. He is the publisher of AdventureKEEN and resides with his family in Birmingham, Alabama.

DEAR CUSTOMERS AND FRIENDS,

SUPPORTING YOUR INTEREST IN OUTDOOR ADVENTURE, travel, and an active lifestyle is central to our operations, from the authors we choose to the locations we detail to the way we design our books. Menasha Ridge Press was incorporated in 1982 by a group of veteran outdoorsmen and professional outfitters. For many years now, we've specialized in creating books that benefit the outdoors enthusiast.

Almost immediately, Menasha Ridge Press earned a reputation for revolutionizing outdoors- and travel-guidebook publishing. For such activities as canoeing, kayaking, hiking, backpacking, and mountain biking, we established new standards of quality that transformed the whole genre, resulting in outdoor-recreation guides of great sophistication and solid content. Menasha Ridge Press continues to be outdoor publishing's greatest innovator.

The folks at Menasha Ridge Press are as at home on a whitewater river or mountain trail as they are editing a manuscript. The books we build for you are the best they can be, because we're responding to your needs. Plus, we use and depend on them ourselves.

We look forward to seeing you on the river or the trail. If you'd like to contact us directly, visit us at menasharidge.com. We thank you for your interest in our books and the natural world around us all.

SAFE TRAVELS,

Bob Sehlinger

BOB SEHLINGER
PUBLISHER